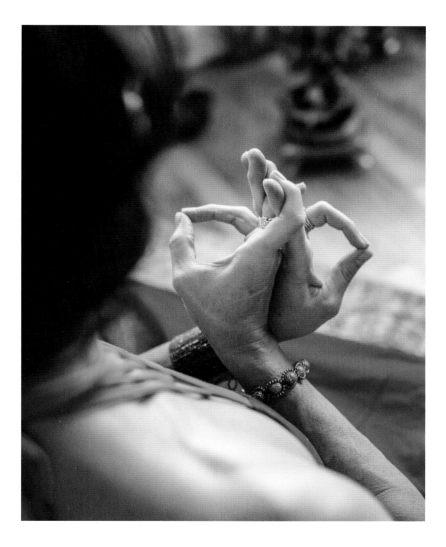

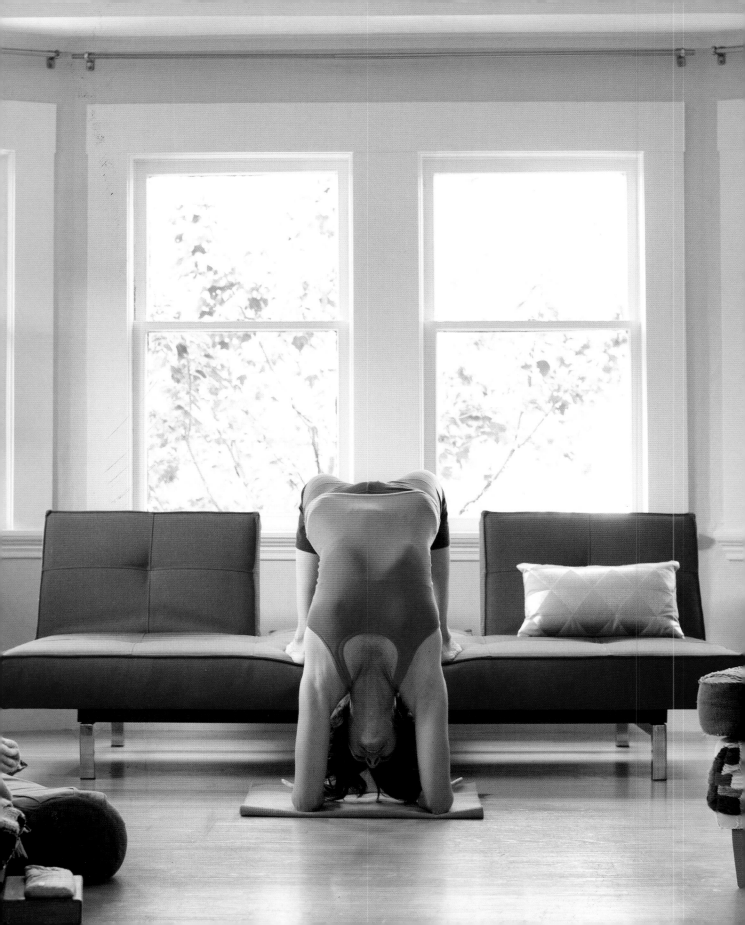

YOGA
AT HOME

Inspiration for
Creating Your Own
Home Practice

LINDA SPARROWE

Photography by
SARAH KEOUGH

UNIVERSE | YOGA JOURNAL

CONTENTS

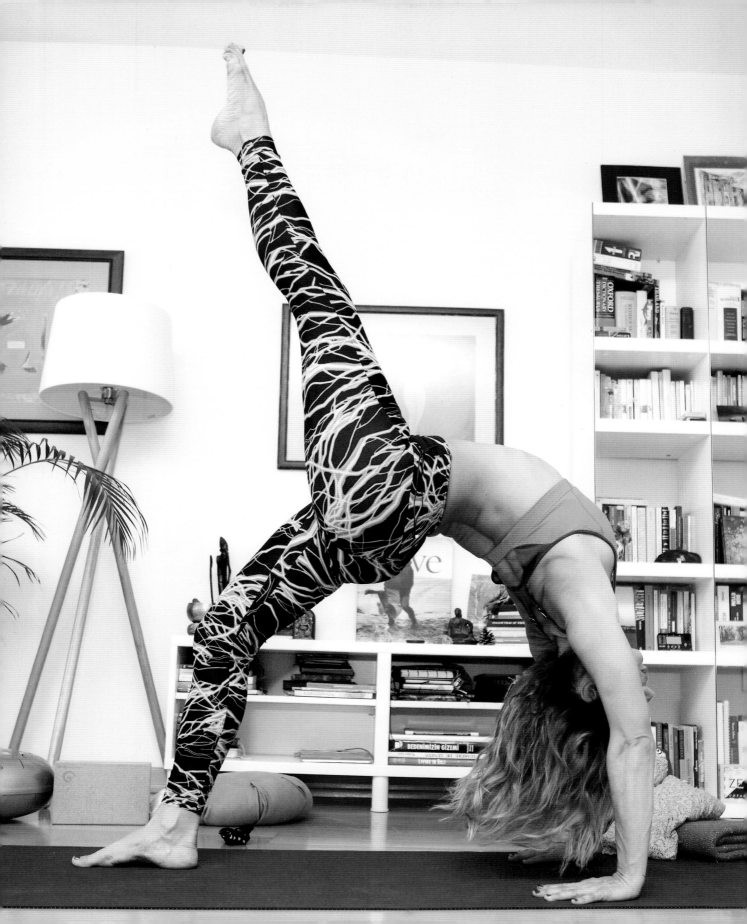

INTRODUCTION

For the first few years after I started doing yoga, I struggled with my home practice. Even though I understood the benefits, I still couldn't make myself do it on a regular basis. *Maybe the space isn't serious enough*, I thought, so I outfitted a whole room in my house, complete with an altar (on my dad's old army trunk) where I placed photos of my teachers and my family; a beloved eighteenth-century Buddha with tiny scrolls of scripture embedded in his wooden spine; and a small porcelain vase a friend's mother had wanted me to have just before she died. I also added a little rice-paper-and-wrought-iron box that houses four wooden teeth a Tibetan friend gave me, which he said were made from the Buddha's own teeth (you can tell because they have mantras etched into them), and a small glass jar with a scoop of sand the Dalai Lama's monks let me have back in the early 1990s before they swept the Kalachakra sand mandala they had made into a river ("What part of impermanence do you not understand, Linda?"). I brought in blocks and bolsters, a couple blankets, a few straps, and an assortment of other props to accompany my well-worn yoga mat.

But when I stepped onto my mat, I still couldn't think of a thing to do. I struggled to remember sequences and wondered whether backbends came before forward bends or if doing a twist too soon would somehow screw up my spine or leave me agitated the rest of the day. *Did I really just move into Downward-Facing Dog and forget to flow through my vinyasa properly? Maybe I should start again.* And then there were days when all I wanted to do was lie in Savasana or do some restoratives, but I didn't because I was afraid I hadn't done enough energizing poses to deserve to rest. Most days, I would get frustrated and end up doing pranayama instead, meditating for a while, and then brewing myself a cup of tea.

In my desire to do things exactly right, I had somehow missed the point of home practice: it's personal. How could it be otherwise when its purpose is to cultivate an intimate relationship between the body and the mind through the agency of the breath; to cut through the noise and reconnect us with our true essence, our basic goodness? Instead, I had forged a rather tenuous union that was more like taking dancing lessons with a blind date—awkward and confusing, with plenty of missteps and then surprising moments of rhythmic connection. I wanted that dance teacher (in reality, my yoga teacher) not only to teach me the steps, but also to create the magic that would ensure a joyous and long-lasting relationship. I wanted one sequence I could do every single day to become a stronger, kinder, and more spiritual person. Of course, I somehow neglected to notice that all the meditating and pranayama I was doing—because I couldn't figure out how to practice yoga—was in fact my home practice.

Since then, I've discovered that I'm not the only one who was confused. A lot of practitioners get tripped up believing that home practice has to be a reflection of what goes on in a yoga class. I really thought that if I didn't have 90 minutes, or at least an hour, to devote to yoga—and by yoga I mean a set routine of poses—then I shouldn't do anything. Surprisingly, this isn't just a newbie problem. Seasoned practitioners and even yoga teachers have their own refrains of resistance—*I don't have time, I have no space of my own, I don't have any idea what to do, I teach so I don't need it.* But the desire to strengthen the relationship between the mind and the body, the body-mind and the heart, remains

---

Linda Sparrowe spends an inordinate amount of time in her home studio, where she uses all sorts of props to personalize her practice.

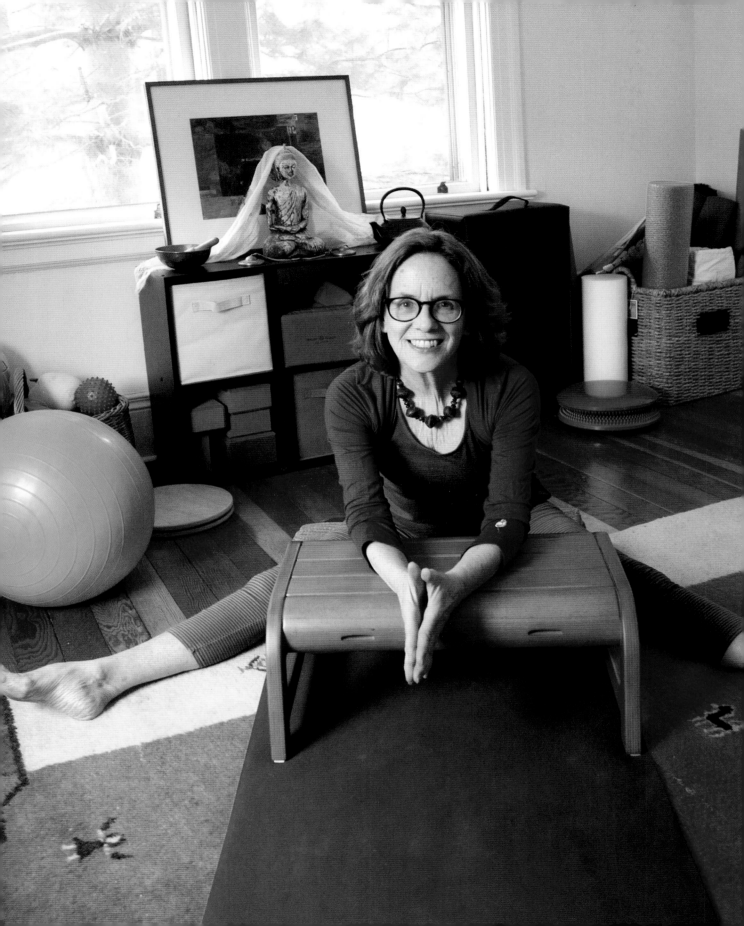

strong. While pretty much everyone agrees that there's no better way to get to know ourselves than to take yoga home with us, not everyone agrees about how to do it.

When I asked Rodney Yee, codirector of Yoga Shanti in New York (and Gaiam TV superstar), why we should practice at home, he answered, "Why home practice? I think it's *only* home practice. You go to class to get ideas, hear another voice, break open another way of seeing something." But without home practice, "you have no way to digest it," he says. Without making it your own, "it doesn't mean anything. Then it's just an exercise class."

While many of us have wonderful "aha" moments in class, practicing at home can take us deeper. It removes all the distractions and invites us to listen to who we are and what we need—at this moment, with this breath. It's not a matter of what we look like to other people, what we hope to be or what we fear we've become. In the privacy of our own space, in the intimacy of our own mind, we can witness the dance going on inside of us and choose the music and create the steps necessary to join in.

In *Yoga at Home*, you'll come to see—through photographs of and interviews with more than fifty yoga and meditation practitioners—that the dances and steps vary widely. Hopefully, this book will broaden your definition of what home practice really is. These men and women invited us into their homes

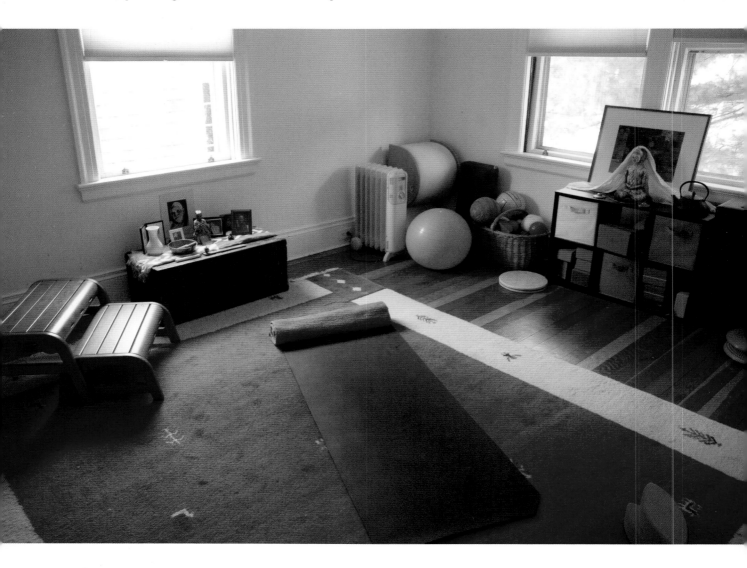

and spoke freely about their practices: both specific rituals and seemingly mundane activities, their lives on the mat and in the real world. Some of the people we interviewed, like jazz saxophonist Sonny Rollins, say they don't do so much yoga anymore. And yet, everything Sonny does is imbued with his love for and connection with the Divine. To enter into his home is to enter into sacred space. Others break out into yoga poses every chance they get. Richard Freeman does his full practice in his yoga room, but considers his whole house to be one big yoga prop that allows him to spontaneously bust a yoga move in any room, even halfway up the stairs.

Some practitioners have created sacred spaces elaborately outfitted with meaningful photos, statues, and mementos that remind them that their "practice is actually in service of others," as Mary Taylor suggests. Others carve out space wherever they can find it—the corner of a laundry room or a converted pantry in a tiny studio kitchen.

You'll see many inspiring examples of different places to practice. Of course, you'll also discover ways in which personal practice extends beyond the mat or the cushion, becoming deeply entwined with and informing everyday life. Cooking meals for friends, feeding the birds in the morning, or preparing breakfast for rescue cats—all this is *seva* (service) and part of daily practice.

Regardless of how each one of these contributors defines personal practice, one teaching emerges loud and clear: it's not so much what you do but the intention you set, the purpose you bring to your action that makes it a "practice." Your ability to listen to what is really needed. Tias Little says, "Home practice is how we till the soil of our body-mind and plant the seeds for a contemplative practice," the way we can discover who we really are right now, not who we hope to be or who we try to be for the benefit of others.

So, enjoy this book. Allow it to inspire you, give you new ways of looking at practice, and, ultimately, free you from the tyranny of exactitude and expectations.

❧

Linda Sparrowe made her dad's old army trunk into an altar that houses items and photos that remind her of why she practices in the first place.

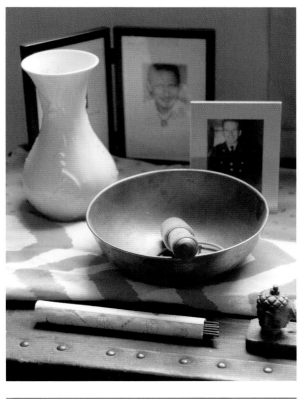

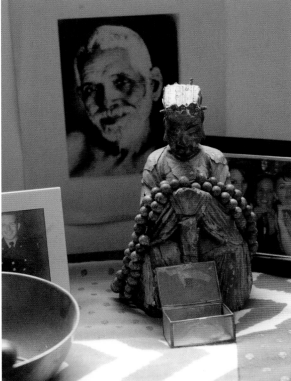

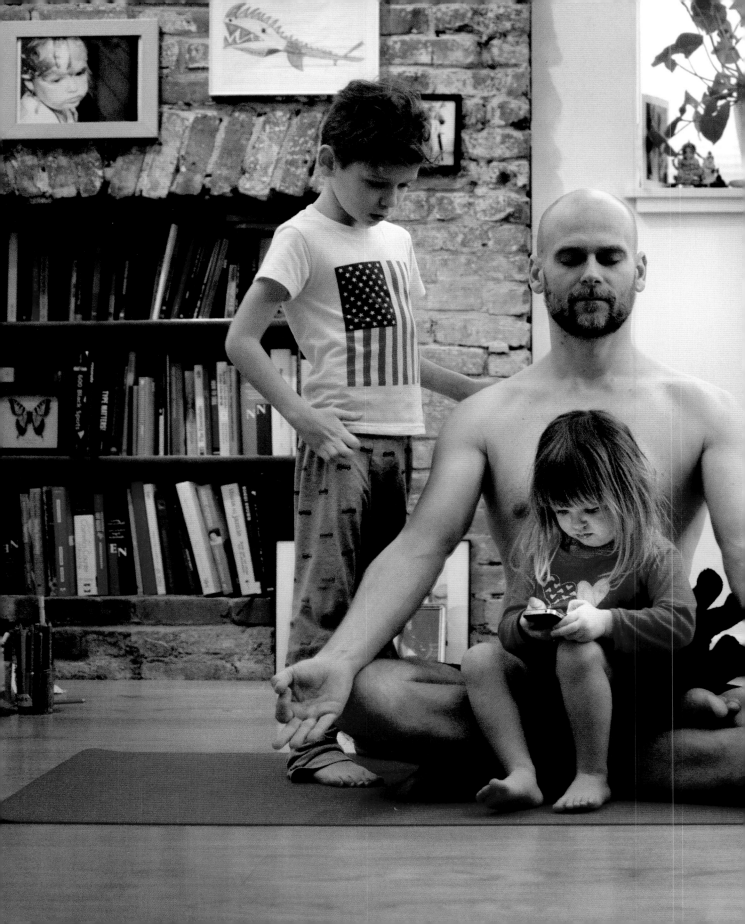

"My goal is to get up at 6:15 a.m. during the week to do 30 minutes of yoga. It is far from a tranquil or meditative type of yoga, because most of the time my kids are awake and trying to climb on top of me while I'm going from Upward-Facing to Downward-Facing Dog."

Bas Van Koll

SANTA BARBARA, CALIFORNIA | CREATIVE DIRECTOR

SPACE

One of the biggest challenges of creating a consistent home practice is finding space—in your home and in your mind—to actually do it. You might be fortunate enough to have a dedicated room in which you can spread out your mat, place your props at the ready, and construct an altar or put some shelves up to hold items of special significance. If you're really lucky, you might even have another smaller room outfitted just for meditation and reflection. Conversely, you might live in a tiny place and have just enough space to turn around in without colliding with the kitchen counter or the couch/pull-out bed in the living room/dining room/bedroom combo. Or, perhaps a more peripatetic practice suits you better, so you can choose the bedroom when the morning light streams in and move onto the deck as day becomes evening and the sunset is too spectacular to ignore. Regardless of what you have available, you can still imbue the space (or multiple spaces) with qualities that can ground and inspire you and keep you coming back to the mat, even on those days you'd rather not.

❦ FINDING PHYSICAL SPACE

Before you carve out a mat's worth of real estate in the hallway or the laundry room, or embark on a whole room remodel, make sure the space you have in mind will work for you—which essentially means you can picture yourself practicing there. As you survey the situation, ask yourself these questions:

❦ How Public Is Your Practice?

In other words, if you like surrounding yourself with reminders of "real" life and can, in the middle of it all, tune out and drop in, then by all means put your mat down in your busy family room. On the other hand, if you easily get distracted or annoyed by constant interruptions, a quieter, more secluded spot (with a door you can close) may work better.

❦ Does the Space Give You What You Need?

If you don't have the luxury of keeping your mat rolled out at all times, is there a closet available nearby to stash it between sessions or a corner where you can

---

SUSAN KRAFT
My Heart-Filled Space

When my daughter Stella left home, I moved my yoga practice into her bedroom. I imagined my new space as pure serenity, but soon gave up on that fantasy. The walls I painted a springtime green ended up a popsicle lime. I also realized that I couldn't possibly paint over the "fresco" that her pal Smurfo had created in her honor during high school. I love having that reminder of her in the room as I practice, and I especially love that it is a reminder of one of the more challenging times to be her mom. We moved a fair amount when Stella was growing up, but any space she has ever occupied feels like home to me. And home, I believe, is what practice should feel like.

An altar and two zafus fit snugly into a small alcove where Rodney Yee and Colleen Saidman-Yee can face one another and begin their day by practicing pranayama.

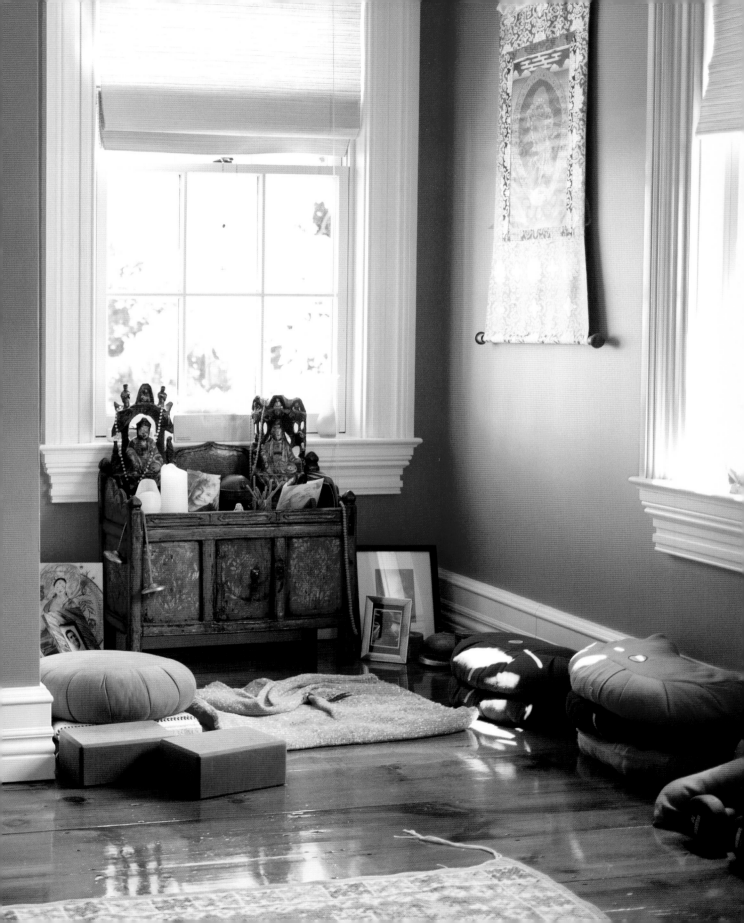

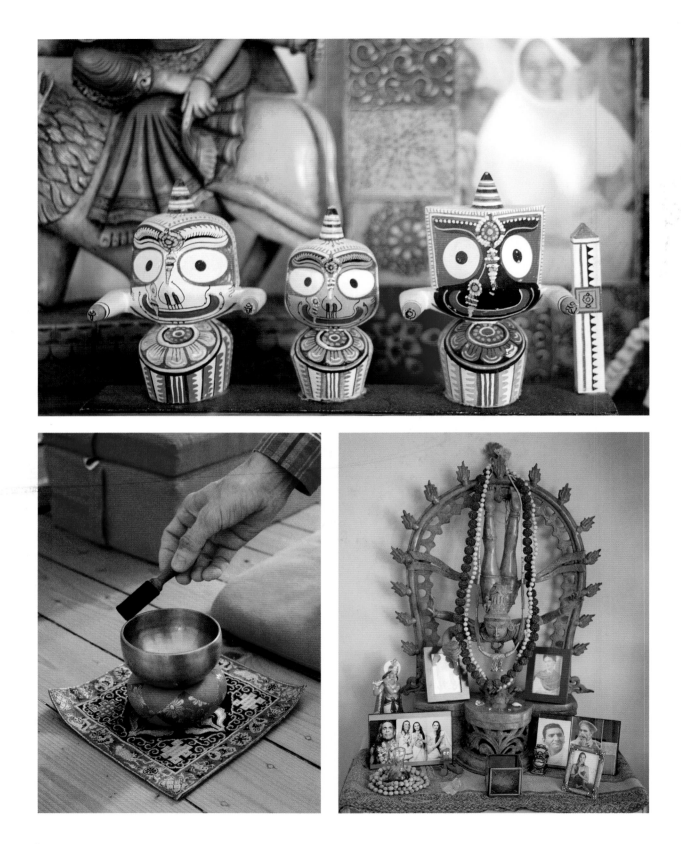

hide a basket full of props? Does your space have an unadorned wall for inversions or restorative poses or a little bookcase for your inspirational books?

☽ Is the Space More Available at Certain Times?

If you love meditating in a tiny alcove off the kitchen, you may need to schedule your practice at odd hours when no one else is in there cooking, eating, or tidying up. If you live with roommates, negotiate certain times of the day to use the study or living room for practice.

❧ CARING FOR YOUR SPACE

Regardless of how tiny a space you have, or how multipurpose it is, you can organize it in a way that creates a sense of spaciousness and gives it the attention it deserves. Get rid of anything you no longer need or that no longer serves the purpose of your newly created space by recycling papers, donating books or clothing, or having a garage sale. Once you feel satisfied, set the intention to keep that area clean and orderly. As Cyndi Lee, founder of OM Yoga in New York City, says, we are in a relationship with everything, including inanimate objects—every book, pillar, and lamp in our space. Organizing your physical space is not about creating rituals or doing anything extraordinary, she says, it's a way to "stay engaged with the things of your life in a wakeful and meaningful way." Such precise attention creates clarity and spaciousness. The more welcoming the space is, the more enthusiastic the mind will be to show up. And the more you practice there, the more sacred the space will feel. It won't take long before just walking by that hallway or setting foot in that laundry room (or your big, beautiful yoga room) will deepen your desire to practice.

❧ CREATING SACRED SPACE

Once the space is free of clutter and chaos, you can organize it in a way that defines it as your yoga space. If you can't have everything you need out and available at all times, choose a few special things that you can keep in a cupboard or bins and pull them out when you're ready to practice. You can even make a simple, removable altar to set them on. All of this will remind you to take your seat, as the yogis say, with the

ALICIA BARRY
The Energy of My Room

When I place myself on my mat in my yoga space, which used to be my daughter's room, I am bathed in memories of how fragile and unsure I was as a young mother, my many vulnerable and laughable attempts to figure things out, the steady climb toward spiritual healing that helped me grow my "mother bones," and the gratitude I feel in becoming the confident and joy-filled mother and woman I longed to be.

I didn't have a mother, so when my daughter Jordan was born, I wanted to be the one person in her life who would love her unconditionally. And that's exactly what I did, even though I was afraid, even though I felt inadequate, even though I had no one to learn from.

In this room, I would rock her, dance with her, sing to her, read to her, and lie with her as she fell asleep. As she grew up and we went through the many stages of childhood and adolescence, I would sit at the end of her bed and listen to the challenges and triumphs of her days. She is now thirty-one years old and happily married. We are truly best friends. In this room, I continue to practice, bathed in the presence of our love.

intention to pay attention for a few breaths or even a couple of hours.

For Sharon Gannon, cofounder of Jivamukti Yoga in New York City, intention is key. "Sacred space is created when someone sees it as such," she says. "You can make a fire hydrant or a parking lot sacred if you're willing to invest in that space." Divinity comes from within you, so creating sacred space, she says, is just

Choosing elements that have special meaning for you will help bring a sense of the sacred to whatever space you create.

JULES FEBRE
It's All Sacred

Creating a sacred space has become a saying that yogis use often and it can mean so many different things. My brother and I turned the word *sacred* into an acronym: Sanctifying And Creating Reality Every Day. In other words, all spaces are sacred if I have the good sense to remember. It starts with honoring my parents and my teachers, and giving thanks to everything that brought me to where I am. When I see the events of my life and myself as worthy of being sacred, then the space around me automatically becomes sacred.

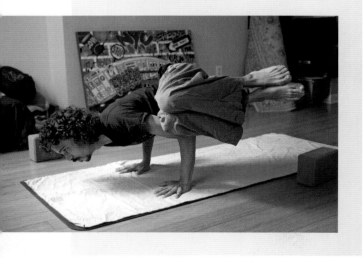

practice, a sense of seriousness or determined effort (what the ancient yogis called *tapas*). Still others feel that concrete elements—from a simple vase of flowers to an elaborate altar full of photos, mementos, sacred objects, and statues—help them dive a little deeper. Most everyone agrees that doing yoga at home brings a sense of divine energy to the whole house and imbues its inhabitants with a little more mindful attentiveness.

For James Brown, a bicoastal yoga teacher from Los Angeles, it's not the room at all, or even its contents, that makes the space sacred. It's the practice that happens there. The space, ideally, provides a container for practice, he says, that "doesn't get in the way of the practice itself." Sure, it's great to have everything you need all in one dedicated, single-purpose space, but "fortunately," says James, "it's not required."

BRENDA FEUERSTEIN
Creating Sacred Space

My small meditation room is screened off with a beautiful Balinese screen that was a gift from one of my students. That space is clearly defined and people don't wander into it. My main practice room where I dance; do yoga poses, pranayama, and yoga nidra; chant; and sing is much bigger and is covered with *thangkas* (Buddhist paintings). I encourage people to wander into the space to get a feeling of peacefulness—especially if they arrive at my home feeling anxious. In some ways, it's a healing space because the space itself tends to have that effect on people and animals.

I create the sacredness of the space by the act of stepping into it. I guess any space could be sacred because I set that intention when I consciously and mindfully enter into it. I do, however, keep my practice space more precious by saying mantras when I enter it, even during nonpractice times. In the evening, I create a deeper kind of sacredness by having the lights out or having lit candles in various areas.

"taking some of that sacredness from your own soul and sprinkling the fairy dust wherever you want."

For some practitioners, simply stepping onto their mat or even just the act of rolling it out signals their commitment to practice. For others, the daily ritual of preparing the space—cleaning the area and lighting candles or incense—prepares the mind. Showing up on purpose brings an element of the sacred into the

Brenda Feuerstein's small meditation room contains an elaborate altar and special ritual items she uses for her Tibetan Buddhist practice.

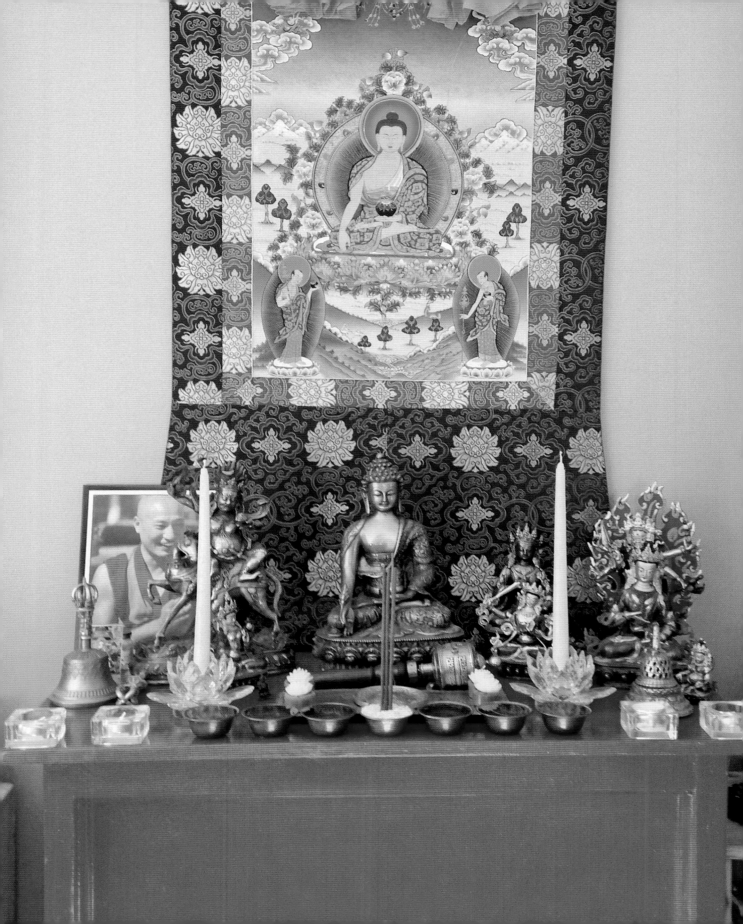

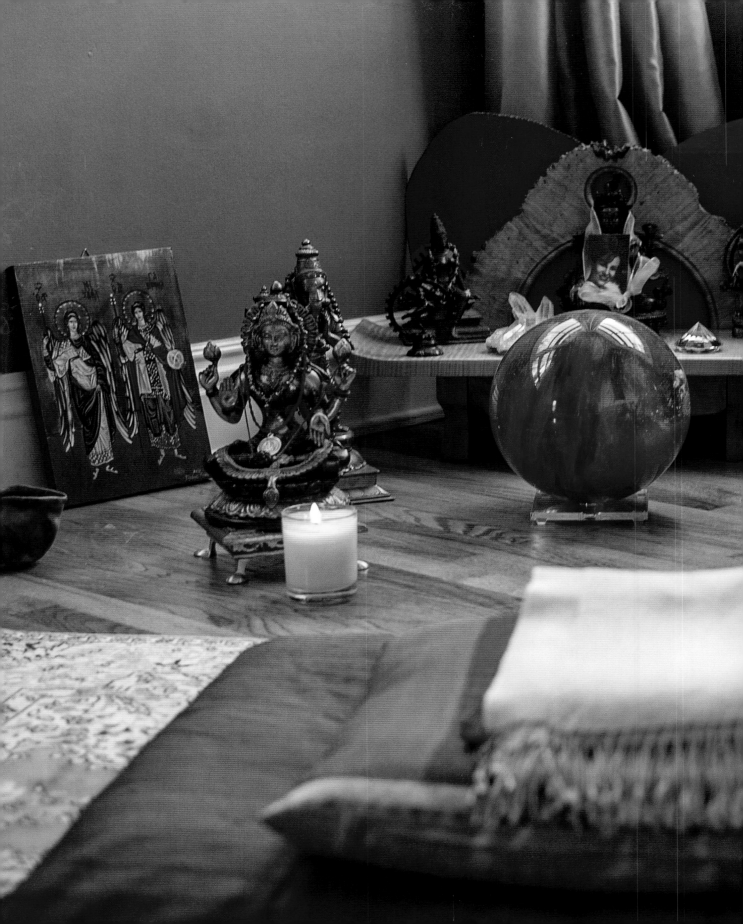

❧ CREATING MENTAL SPACE

Of course, carving out physical space sometimes is the least of our concerns. Finding space in our day and in our mind to actually practice, even in the most perfect home yoga space imaginable, can prove to be the biggest stumbling block of all. The following respected yoga teachers offer suggestions to help you get out of your own way and onto the mat.

JAMES BROWN

Prioritize your practice in your ongoing daily schedule. That's the number one thing that gets me there. Nothing works better for me than a nonnegotiable time slot. If I've designated a chunk of time where practice is the only allowed activity, I get on the mat and see what happens.

BRENDA FEUERSTEIN

Dedicate your practice to someone other than yourself, someone in need. Knowing that I do my practice to help others makes it very real in a big way and helps me look past my excuses.

GISELLE MARI

Crank up the tunes. I use music as my persuader because it encourages me to move. Before I know it, I've shimmied my way to the mat and—voilà!—instant Sun Salutation. And then, of course, one thing leads to another.

SIANNA SHERMAN
Using Sacred Objects

My home *sadhana* (practice) space is my temple. The altars, *murtis* (images of the Divine Spirit), spiritual paintings, *thangkas* (Buddhist paintings), books, and musical instruments I've put there remind me of the divine energies of life. My sadhana temple is decorated with sacred art and photos of lineage teachers and saints. But in truth, I consider our entire home to be sacred space.

LINNEA VEDDER
Anywhere Spaces

The space I have created for my home practice has defined the vibe of my entire living space. Residing in a small apartment in Brooklyn is a lot like living on a boat, where everything and every room serves multiple functions. I practice yoga in my living room, where we have a big white sofa, a soft Persian rug, tons of plants, and art that my partner, our friends, and I have made. I can use the tile floor for my standing poses and move onto the carpet to practice meditation or supine poses.

DESIREE RUMBAUGH

Practice without a goal or destination in mind. I get on my mat solely for the purpose of feeling better. Who wouldn't want to feel better? Think of it as playtime and work time all rolled into one.

KAITLIN QUISTGAARD

Rather than sanctifying a corner for yoga, we live as consciously as possible everywhere. I can unfurl my mat on the deck, in our bedroom, or in the living room and just connect with the practice.

SINEM ER

Step onto your mat. I stand in Tadasana for some time, feeling the ground, the air, and my body, or I just sit down and meditate. After some time, my body starts moving. Or not. Once I figure out what I need, I get to it. Sometimes this means sitting to practice some pranayama and meditation, or jotting down a few thoughts. Regardless of what I actually do, if it's an expression of what is alive in me, then that practice helps me stay present.

❧ ——————————————

Some practitioners, like Sianna Sherman, use sacred art, statuary, and photos of their teachers and saints as a way to infuse their practice space with the divine energies of life.

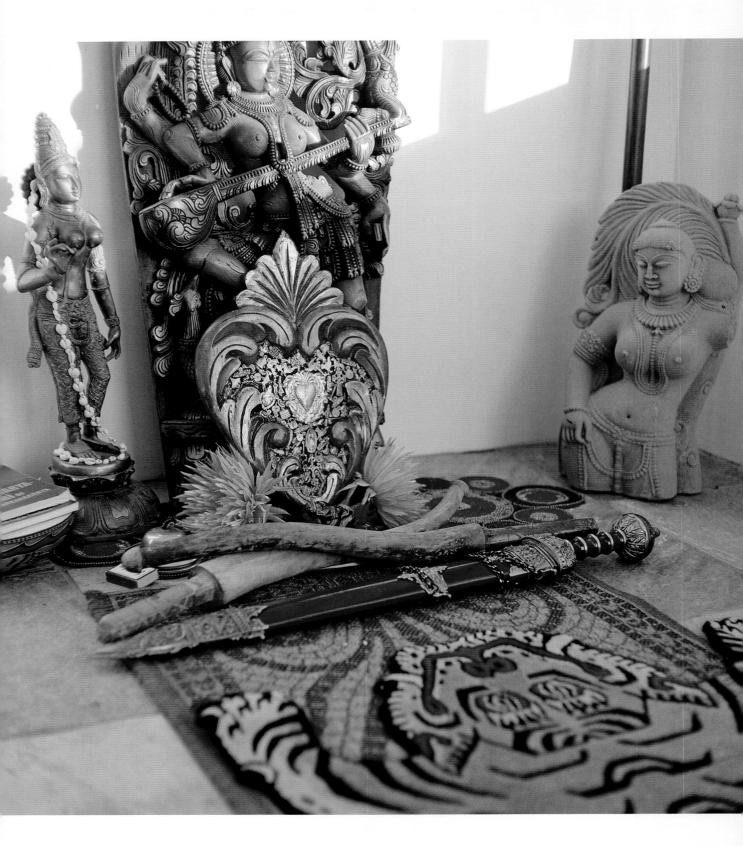

Shiva Rea's
Create Your Own Altar

Any place can be a living altar. The *Bhagavad Gita* implores us to offer every action—the beautiful, the fragmented, and the difficult—back to the source. Your altar is the space that allows you to "come as you are," that offers you 365 days of acceptance as well as the power to change, renew, ignite, and dissolve.

From a simple flower you lay lovingly on the front of your mat to a candle or a picture of your beloved to a more elaborate shrine with statuary, tapestries, and beads, altars can be a way to invoke the sacred and connect the personal to the universal. Even if chaos, clutter, or disarray is all around (or inside) you, you can still bring loving attention, creativity, and, most of all, your own joy to your altars.

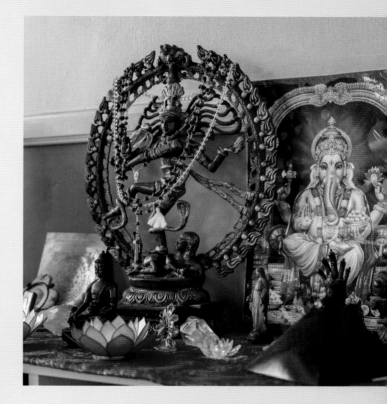

☙ CHOOSE YOUR SPACE

Your personal altar connects your inner and outer worlds and acts as a conduit for your creative energy and prayers; it is a reflection of your inner process. So choose a place that truly speaks to you—inside or outside of your home. Look to nature for inspiration.

☙ PURIFY YOUR SACRED SPACE

Honor the sacred space by regularly cleaning and refreshing it. Clear away any objects that may have outlived their purpose. Remove dust, wilted flowers, or ashes and wax left from burning incense and candles. You can bathe sacred objects in water, or dust them with a special cloth that you only use for your altar. You can do this daily or weekly, each time invoking a new beginning connected to this symbolic ritual of revival.

☙ PERSONALIZE YOUR ALTAR

Place your central symbols on an altar cloth made of any natural material of any color. Have several cloths on hand and change them whenever it feels appropriate—during the *sadhana* (practice), on special occasions, or in accordance with the lunar cycles.

☙ BRING IT ALL TOGETHER

Place the cloth on the altar and fill the space with colors, using flowers, candles, and juicy fruits that enhance the beauty of your home and fill your home, body, and heart with *rasa* (pure essence).

Continue to enrich your altar with images that speak to you. These can be images of your connection to the sacred source, photos of your family and your teachers, mandalas, aspects of nature that connect you to the seasons or moon cycles—anything that brings a sense of creative power to your process.

☙ ACTIVATE YOUR ALTAR

There are many ways to breathe life into your altar. You can follow your own tradition or a specific *puja* (offering to the deity). At a minimum, sprinkle a little water in each of the four directions, light your candle, circle some incense, and then dedicate your practice for the benefit of all sentient beings.

TOOLS & PROPS

For years, yoga props were mostly used by Iyengar teachers or yoga therapists as a way to help students benefit from poses their bodies couldn't do on their own—maybe because they were ill or injured, pregnant, too old, or simply new to the practice. Other styles of yoga rarely encouraged students to use props; the stigma associated with doing so relegated such tools to "beginners' necessities." As a consequence, you'd only reach for a strap or grab a block if you weren't flexible enough to hold your feet in a Seated Forward Bend or touch the floor in poses like Triangle or Side Angle Pose. Even then the goal, of course, was to eventually be able to shed those external reminders of how stiff or weak you were.

These days, just about every yoga studio in town has at least a wall unit or a whole closet full of mats, bolsters, blocks, straps, and blankets; a basket of eye bags; and plenty of unadorned wall space. Iyengar studios make room for all of that, and add in a couple dozen straight-backed chairs in a light gray, shiny metal; a bunch of dangling ropes securely fastened along a reinforced wall; cloth-covered, ten-pound sandbags; and a collection of wooden backbenders with varying degrees of curvature. Other studios have scarves hanging from the ceiling, slings, swings, resistance straps bolted to the wall, and balls of all sizes and degrees of squishiness. Whole classes are devoted to being suspended from those scarves, hanging from those ropes, or rolling those balls along the spine, neck, inner thighs, and feet.

Obviously, this is far too much paraphernalia to fit in your home practice space unless you're fortunate enough to have a dedicated room large enough to hold it all. Let's take a look at the various types of props available and determine what you should have at the ready and what you can do without.

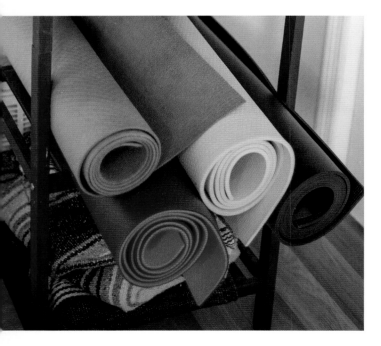

❧

Using props allows us to take the struggle out of our practice and simply notice what is possible at this moment.

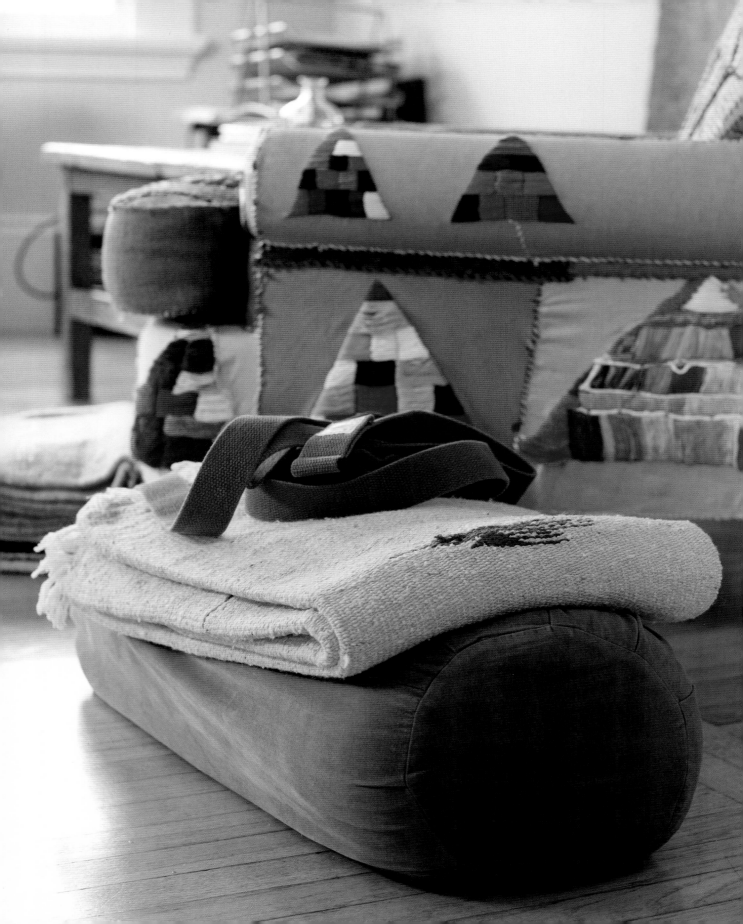

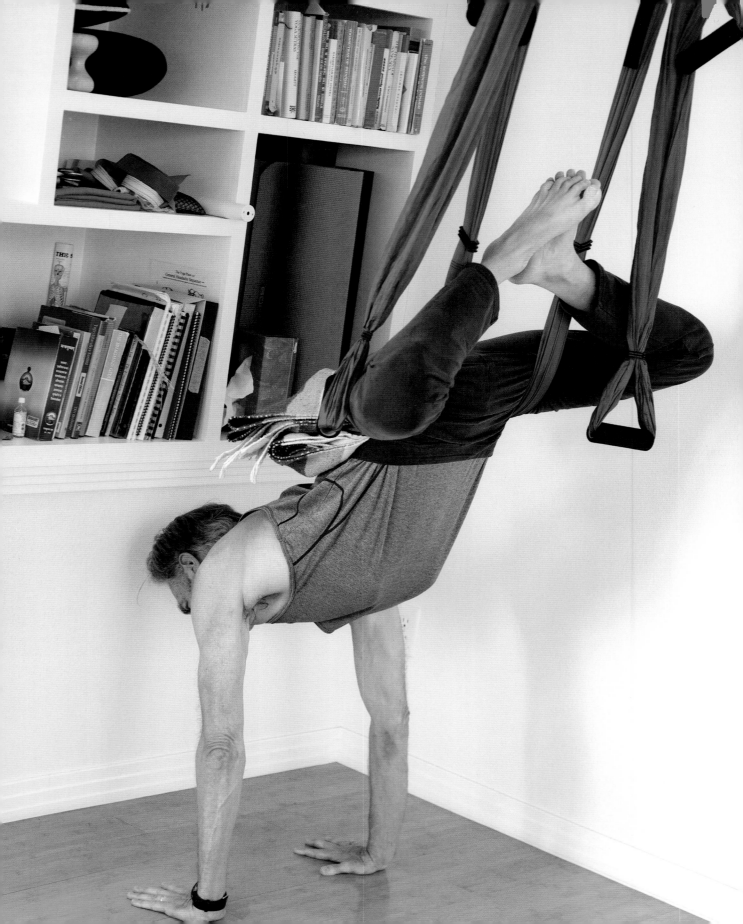

❧ YOUR PROPS CLOSET

Almost anything can be a prop—tables, walls, doorknobs, the kitchen counter, couch cushions, neckties, or a friend's outstretched hand. With so many kinds of props to choose from, you may want to focus on a few essentials first and then branch out to more specialized options depending on your body's needs and the space you have available. Of course, what one person considers a luxury another person may deem essential. But for the most part, props like mats, blocks, straps, blankets, and bolsters are nonnegotiable must-haves in your props closet, while backbenders, body lifts for headstands, and yoga slings attached to the ceiling might end up on your wish list. Here are descriptions of the more common props and some suggestions on how to use them.

MATS

Luckily, the choice of yoga mats has broadened considerably in the last few years. Gone are the days when the only choice was to press your face into a yoga mat made of PVC, a type of plastic that has been softened by phthalates (plasticizers)—known carcinogens and endocrine disruptors—and then stabilized with lead and cadmium. PVC does put the sticky in sticky mats and makes them spongy and soft, but at a great environmental cost.

Alternatives are getting better. Some mats are made from PER (polymer environmental resin), which is a more sustainable material. Several companies make mats out of natural rubber or recycled tires; others combine natural rubber and jute to make mats that you can compost in the garden when you're through with them; and still others hark back to the days when yogis practiced on grass mats or rugs woven in cotton (organic, of course). None of the alternatives boasts the stickiness of PVC, but washing your mat before use (and hanging it to dry) should help. The nubbier, raised texture of some of the cotton mats will also prevent you from slip-sliding away. If you practice heated vinyasa or Bikram yoga, placing a yoga towel over your mat will help absorb your sweat.

Mats come as thin as ⅟₁₆ inch (good for folding up in a suitcase) and as thick as ¼ inch, for those who need a little extra padding on their bones. Although most mats are about six feet long and two feet wide,

Creative Propping

Don't let the absence of props stop you from getting the support you need in the poses you do. You'll see plenty of examples of creative propping as you thumb through these pages. James Brown uses a big boulder in Central Park to stretch up and over in a backbend; Maya Kanako rests her leg on the edge of her sink for a nice hamstring stretch; Margi Young relies on her bright red couch to make her Bridge Pose a blissfully restorative one; and Jan Schmidt gets a little shoulder-opening assist from her husband, Arthur Rivers.

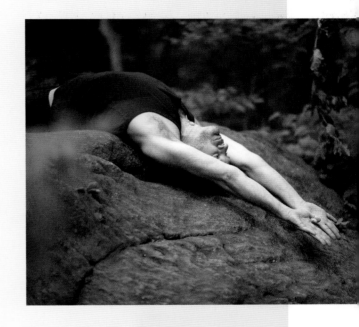

you can find some that extend to eight feet long and three feet wide, some that are six feet square, and even some circular ones that are six feet in diameter.

❧

Richard Freeman has a little fun kicking up into Handstand using a yoga swing suspended from the ceiling.

BLOCKS

Aside from a yoga mat, the most ubiquitous prop is the rectangular block (or brick). You can purchase blocks in a couple of different styles: traditional rectangular ones made of foam, cork, or wood; or oval-shaped foam ones called Three Minute Eggs. Choose the material that feels safest and most comfortable for your purpose. Most blocks are nine inches high, but the thickness can vary—between two and four inches. Some experts suggest that you might prefer the thinner blocks (two or three inches) if you have small hands or if you are more flexible. Pressing against a block can give you more lift through the spine, length in the side body, and more opening in the front body.

- **FOAM BLOCKS** are the lightest and generally the cheapest option and are comfortable to lie over. They won't win any eco-friendly awards, however, so do your homework and search out ones made from recycled foam. The oval-shaped foam blocks come in soft, medium, or hard densities, and some are eco-sourced.
- **CORK BLOCKS** are usually heavier, depending on the density of the foam ones. Some practitioners prefer these because they're more stable, they absorb sweat better than foam, and they tend not to slip on a wood floor. Look for cork harvested from sustainable sources.
- **WOOD BLOCKS** are the heaviest, most stable blocks available, but they're not exactly comfortable to lie on. Bamboo blocks tend to be a little bit lighter and more eco-friendly, but these days more of the traditional wooden blocks come from sustainable forests as well.

BOLSTERS AND CUSHIONS

Oblong or rectangular in shape, these dense, large pillows are a perfect addition to your props closet. You can sit on them to release your pelvis and improve your alignment, lie over them in supported backbends, or extend onto them in a restorative forward bend. Pranayama or breathing bolsters are thinner and narrower than the others; they're nice to sit on, if you need

Besides the usual blocks, bolsters, chairs, and blankets, Iyengar yogis also love backbending props and ballet-bar-like trestles.

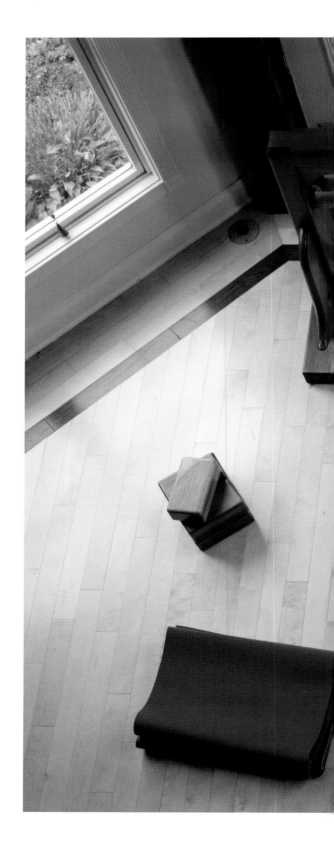

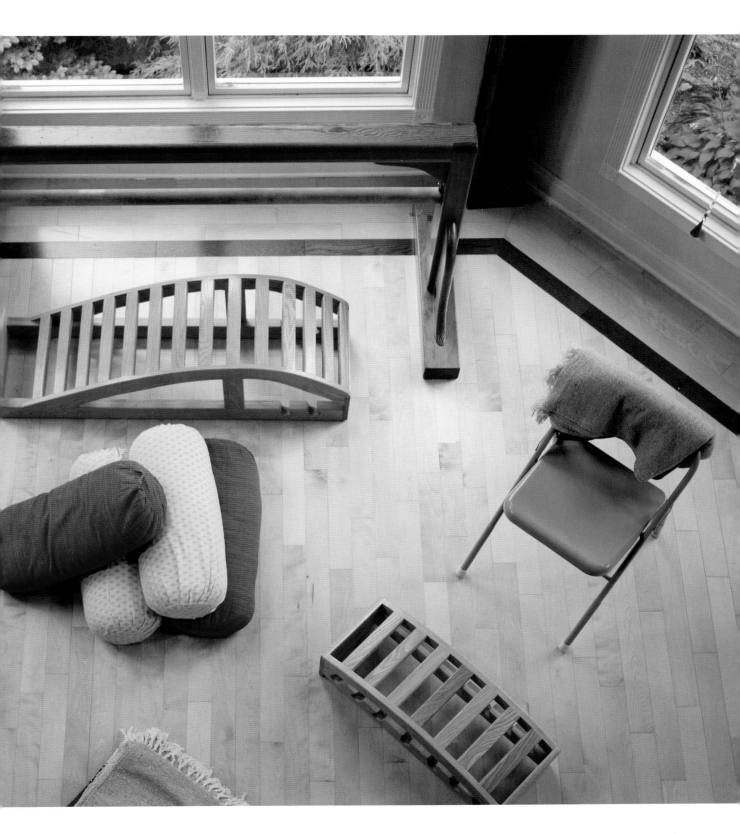

Alternative Tools and Props

Don't have these specific tools and props lying around your house? That's OK! Try these alternatives.

- ❦ **BLOCKS:** If you don't have blocks, you can use anything that provides a hard surface and won't slide out from under you. A large, hardback book (or a stack of books), or even a low bench, works for most poses.

- ❦ **BOLSTERS AND CUSHIONS:** Couch cushions or dense pillows work well in place of bolsters, but bed pillows do not (they're too soft). Two or three yoga blankets trifolded (or two rolled around each other) work better, and they're quite a bit cheaper (and more versatile) than bolsters.

- ❦ **BLANKETS:** You can use regular blankets from home, but they should be slightly stiff, densely woven, and easy to fold. A stack of towels would work in a pinch.

- ❦ **STRAPS:** Good alternatives include two neckties tied together, a bathrobe belt, a long scarf, or a towel.

- ❦ **CHAIRS:** If you don't have the foldable kind, almost any sturdy, straight-backed chair will do.

- ❦ **EYE BAGS AND SANDBAGS:** For eye bags, a folded washcloth can substitute and provide that extra little bit of weight on the eyes to help you relax more. For sandbags, grab a five- or ten-pound bag of rice from your kitchen pantry.

Colleen Saidman-Yee often begins her practice by using blocks to release her stiff shoulders, as she demonstrates here.

less height under your sitting bones, and they support the spine nicely when you lie on them. Choose those that come with removable cotton coverings.

BLANKETS

Cotton or finely woven wool blankets are indispensable in any yoga practice. Placed under your sitting bones, they help keep your spine straight, support your back and neck in supine poses and your neck and head in inversions, and, when rolled up or folded, can take the place of bolsters in restorative poses.

STRAPS

These six-, eight-, or twelve-foot-long cotton straps extend your reach in seated poses and balance poses, and can help organize your arms or legs in inverted poses and standing poses. They're ideal to use in seated forward bends when you need a little more extension to reach your feet. They come in a few different colors and two different widths—skinny and wide—with D rings or black cinch buckles.

CHAIRS

Although chairs are most often found in Iyengar or therapeutic yoga studios, the foldable kind is a great addition to any home practice space. You can use the chair for certain twisting poses, modified backbends, or inversions. If you have limited mobility or are coming off an injury, a whole chair yoga sequence works wonders. Make sure your chair is stable by placing it against the wall and on your sticky mat. And if you use a chair for seated twists, make sure your feet can reach the floor and your thighs are parallel to the floor.

EYE BAGS AND SANDBAGS

Gently weighted eye bags (or eye pillows) can help you relax more and block out external distractions in restorative poses. Sandbags, which usually weigh ten pounds, apply pressure to specific parts of the body. This pressure, similar to a sensory therapy called deep pressure touch stimulation, which is used to reduce anxiety, mimics the feeling of being hugged, swaddled, or massaged. Sandbags feel nice on the small of your back in Balasana (Child's Pose) or on your belly in Savasana (Corpse Pose); they can root your thighs down in Dandasana (Staff Pose) or Upavistha Konasana (Wide-Angle Seated Pose).

WHY USE PROPS?

Unfortunately, some of that prop-as-loser stigma remains in a few styles of yoga and in the minds of more than a few practitioners. But luckily at home no one rolls his eyes at you when you use a prop. Regardless of how advanced you are, no matter what type of yoga you practice, consider experimenting with props; they can support you in several ways.

Props Take the Struggle Away

If you're a newcomer to yoga (or coming back to it after a time away), some poses may seem confusing or even foreign to you. Props can help by decreasing the number of things your body (and mind) has to worry about so you can focus on the mechanics of the pose—where to put your feet, how to extend your arm—and create the length, space, and ease in the body that come with proper alignment. Using conventional props or even a willing partner will help you stay in a pose long enough to notice the stretch in your back leg or the external rotation of your arms and, equally important, the rhythm of your breath and the state of your mind. And once you gain a little confidence, you can experiment with extending more, bending deeper, and breathing more evenly.

This type of support isn't limited to first timers, of course. But sometimes more seasoned practitioners have to remind themselves to lighten up, back off, and slow down. If you've been doing yoga for a long time unassisted, consider using props to find more ease in the poses you already do or to work on some you've never done before.

Props Give the Body Instant Feedback

Both beginning students and longtime practitioners benefit when they can *feel* the pose and understand which muscles need to be activated and which

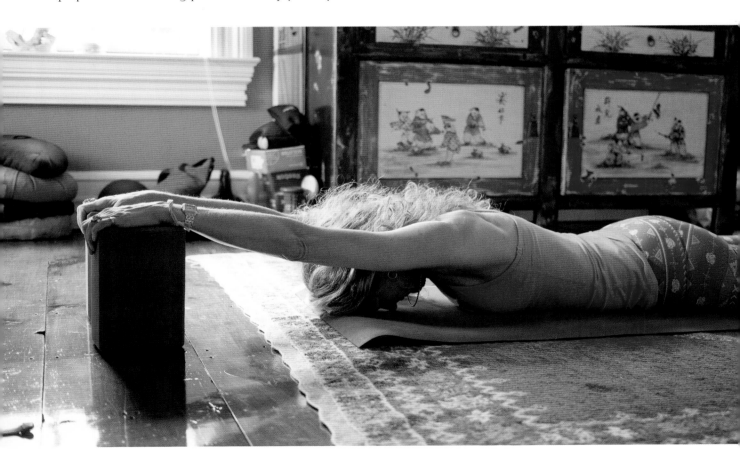

ones can relax. For example, when you put a block between your legs in Utkatasana (Chair Pose), you can tell pretty quickly whether your inner thigh muscles are firing (the block stays in place) or whether they aren't really engaged in the process (the block slips free). By using props, your practice becomes more about listening and less about achieving a goal. And, once you experiment with using props in a particular pose, you can put them aside and try the pose again. Do you notice anything different? Was the feedback helpful? Do you prefer the lift you get from using a block or a strap?

Props Extend Opportunities for Practice

Without props, your yoga practice may be limited to those days when the mind is willing and the body feels strong and capable. What happens when you're tired or anxious, injured, or coming down with a cold? Do you have to shelve your practice until you feel better? Not necessarily. Props allow you to modify and organize poses and sequences to better respond to your physical and emotional needs. By draping yourself over a bolster, for example, you can still benefit from energizing backbends without having to expend a lot of muscular effort.

Props Help Activate the Body's Intelligence

If you ever feel like you're just going through the motions, mindlessly doing your Surya Namaskars (Sun Salutations), standing poses, arm balances, backbends, and twists, you may want to take a break and reach for a few props. Props can move you from autopilot to discrimination, according to B. K. S. Iyengar, and the more you learn to discriminate—to hear and feel what your body is telling you—the more you can discard what contracts or harms and embrace what expands and enlivens.

Maria Rodale stretches her whole body with the help of her Iyengar backbending bench, three bolsters, and a blanket.

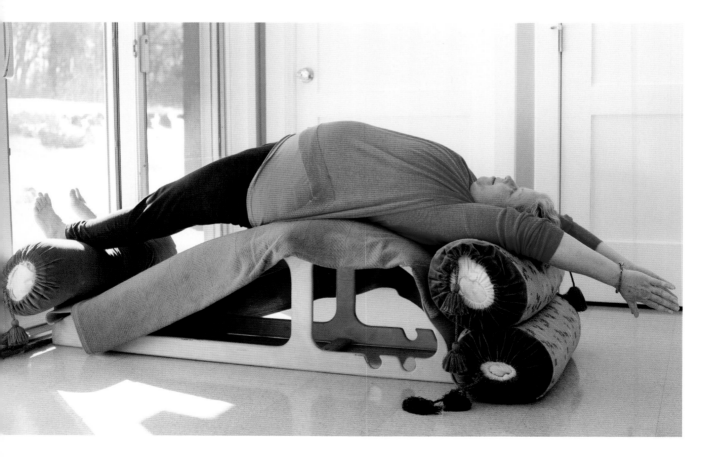

Advancing with Props

MARGI YOUNG

Seeing some of my most advanced students work with props is like a dance between Ginger and Fred. These students possess a thorough knowledge of their physical needs, which may be different every day, and can integrate props mindfully and effortlessly. The blocks glide in just in time for a lunge, the belt appears as if by magic for Gomukhasana (Cow-Face Pose) arms, and, in Savasana, the bolster beautifully offers support under their knees as the eye pillow soothes their eyes.

ANNIE CARPENTER

As the decades pass by in my practice, I find that my love affair with props has only deepened, despite my flexibility and strength. Often, I'll reach for a prop—a block under my hand in Parivrtta Trikonasana (Revolved Triangle Pose), for example—not because I can't reach for the floor, but because I want to know what happens when I take any measure of striving out of the practice. As a longtime practitioner I choose to make the poses as simple as possible so that I can observe my mind without the distraction of physical stress. Clearly this doesn't imply that I am not *working* in this challenging pose. It merely suggests that, thanks to the block, I am able to be steady, strong, and focused, and, at the same time, able to witness my mind wanting to work harder, or run away, or judge ("Nice pose, Annie!" or "After all these years you *still* can't do this?"). Or, on a good day, simply stay present to my calm, steady breathing, feel my feet grounding, legs firming, and spine lengthening and revolving.

To remove the element of striving—of wanting more, ever more—is to invite what we call *sattva*, a harmonious and balanced state. This is the state where one can abide in the truth of the moment, whatever the truth may be. This deeply calming place is where lasting acceptance is tried on and imprinted and, over time, more and more easily returned to even in the most challenging moments.

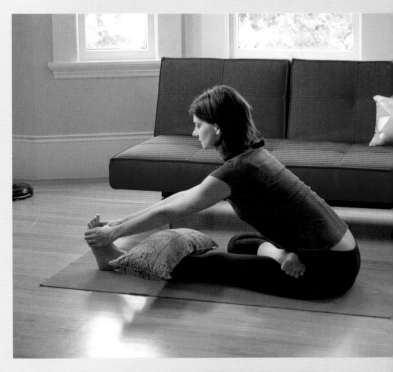

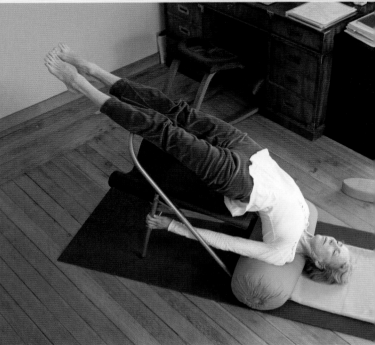

PRACTICE

Once you have your practice space defined, your props picked out and organized, and time carved out of your schedule, you're ready to practice. But practice what exactly?

Luckily, there are no hard-and-fast rules that dictate what you must do, in which order, or for how long. In fact, the only rules I adhere to are what you'd expect from a mindful yoga class: do no harm (*ahimsa*, the Golden Rule of yoga); start your practice where you are (this moment, this breath—not yesterday, not where you hope to be next month); and approach the time on your mat with patience, nonjudgmental curiosity, and generosity. That doesn't mean you can only achieve self-awareness with bolsters and eye bags. A strong, physical practice done mindfully may be just what your body needs. The key is to listen first. Tias Little, creator of Prajna Yoga in Santa Fe, New Mexico, says such a check-in increases somatic awareness, so rather than imposing "a set of sequences onto your body, *a priori*, you can lead a practice that, in the moment, is most appropriate for your physical and mental state."

Of course, you'll find ample, and often seemingly contradictory, advice throughout these pages. Some practitioners believe you should do a set sequence every time you practice; others say it doesn't matter how long you stay on your mat or what you do when you get there—just show up, see what your body needs, and move accordingly. But everyone agrees that personal practice is, well, *personal*. And with guidance from a teacher to get you started, you'll have a container with walls malleable enough to push and pull against until it takes the shape most appropriate to your needs.

Faith Hunter and her darling dogs manage to carve out enough room for all of them to practice in her tiny apartment.

FAITH HUNTER'S
Home Practice

- Stand at the top of your mat, hands resting at your heart. Inhale, feeling the beauty of your life pour in, and then exhale, slowly creating space for abundance. Inhale as you lift your arms overhead, palms touching.

- Exhale forward, step your right foot back for Anjaneyasana (Low Lunge); inhale your arms overhead. Exhale, release your hands, and draw your hips back to stretch your hamstring.

- Inhale, bend your knee, and exhale your right arm to the sky for a spinal twist. Release and step into Adho Mukha Svanasana (Downward-Facing Dog).

- Inhale to Plank Pose, exhale your knees, chest, and chin toward the mat. Slide forward into a low Bhujangasana (Cobra Pose), then shift your hips back into Balasana (Child's Pose).

- Curl your toes under and move into Downward-Facing Dog. Inhale and walk your feet to the top of the mat.

- Breathe in and soften your knees. Roll up to standing and return your hands to your heart. Repeat on the other side.

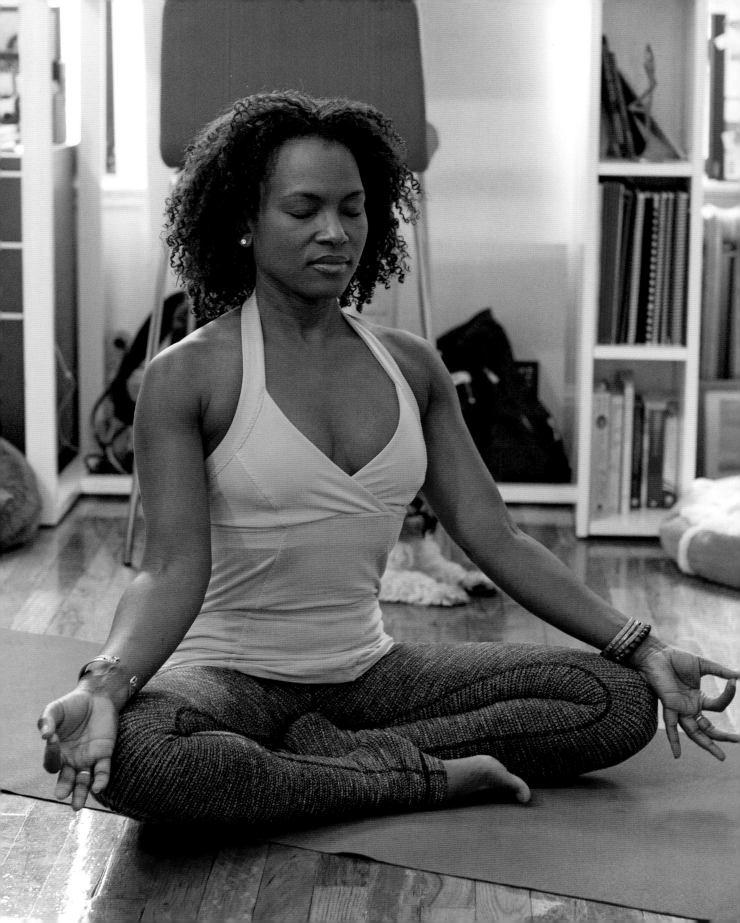

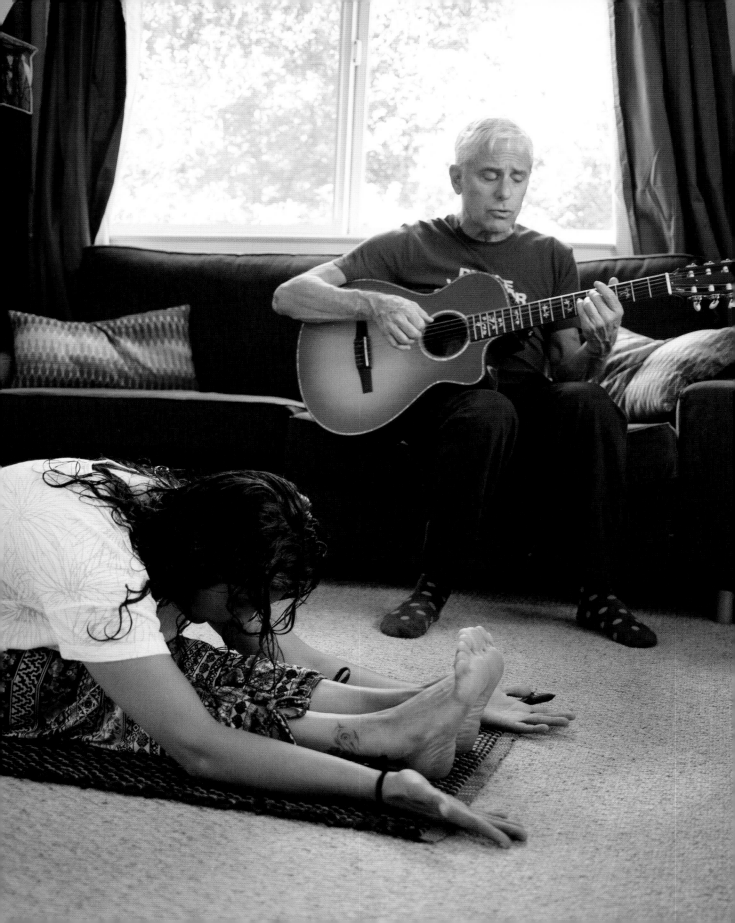

GENERAL GUIDELINES

When thinking about how to structure your own personal practice, it may help to follow these guidelines:

Practice a little every day. Even if you only have 10 or 15 minutes to spare, it's better to do a little bit every day than a 2-hour marathon once every couple of weeks. Gopi Kallayil, the chief evangelist for brand marketing at Google, once told me that he commits to doing 1 minute of yoga and 1 minute of meditation daily. His practice often extends longer, but that's not the point. He always has 2 minutes to spare, he says, 2 minutes to devote to his well-being.

NUBIA TEIXEIRA'S
Good Morning Practice

Stand up with your feet hip-distance apart, and your feet and knees slightly pointing out.

Breathe in as you move your arms upward from the sides, and when you reach the top of your arc, turn your palms skyward.

As you breathe out, bend your knees deeply and move your hands down through the central channel, all the way to the pubic bone. Do three cycles of this breathing, connecting to sky and earth.

Now, squat all the way down into Malasana (Garland Pose), hands in prayer, and focus inward, turning yourself into a beautiful garland to be offered to whomever or whatever represents the sacred to you. Allow all the beauty, aromas, and light to shine.

Press your hands into the earth and lift up to standing.

Walk around in a silent meditation, spreading your goodness and light with each step. And now, take that into your day!

JAI UTTAL'S
Simple Mantra Practice

Sit in your newly created sacred space and light a candle.

Choose a very simple mantra and a very simple melody. Look deep into your heart and find the most vulnerable and yearning part of your being. From that place, sing the mantra for 3 minutes with no expectations or destination.

Bow in gratitude at the end.

Approach your practice with a beginner's mind. No matter how many years you've done yoga, every time you step onto your mat it's a new experience. Cultivate a sense of innocence and simply show up. Set an intention to put aside any preconceived notions of what it means to practice and see if you can embrace your strengths as a gift and your limitations as an adventure.

Acknowledge your limitations, but don't get attached to them. Check in with your body often. Are those limitations still active? If they are, welcome them. But some may come from old fears or outdated habits. Challenge yourself, but balance effort with ease and willpower with compassion.

Be patient. It's always more helpful, and certainly more fun, to approach your practice and your challenges from the perspective of "Isn't that interesting?" instead of "Aren't I awful?"

When you can't practice, get creative. Do some Seated Forward Bends when you watch television or talk to your partner; a few Sun Salutations first thing in the morning while your coffee or tea is brewing; and three rounds of pranayama at the stoplight (but keep your eyes open!).

Jai Uttal and Nubia Teixeira take great delight in practicing together—in every room of their tiny house. Jai's guitar playing and singing fills the room as Nubia does her yoga.

❧ PRACTICE ADVICE

If you struggle to find the time or motivation to commit to a daily practice, don't worry—you're not the only one. Even well-known teachers and longtime practitioners sometimes need help figuring out what, when, and how to practice. Several of them share creative ways to get themselves—and you—on the mat.

INSIYA RASIWALA-FINN

Make your practice a sacred time. Light some incense or a candle before you begin, say an invocation, or chant the Om sound. Perhaps you have a small bowl of beautiful flowers or a deity that you connect with, such as Ganesha or Shiva. Have an assortment of objects on your altar that hold meaning and power and somehow symbolize who you are.

ANNIE CARPENTER

Grab some time. Say you've got 15 minutes. Get on that mat. And then ask yourself: How am I doing and what do I need to feel better? That's all: How am I doing and what do I need? And then follow it. Take one extra minute and make notes on what worked. And then, the next time you show up, do it again. You make it better, you make it different, you increase it, and then you see if it worked.

CYNDI LEE

For a long time, I was influenced by other people's ideas about yoga—ideas like you need to practice every single day for at least an hour and a half, and you need to include this one thing or this other thing. I struggled to do all that and felt guilty when I didn't. I'm older now and I've had a couple of injuries, so finally I've taken my own advice: practice isn't practice until it's personal. It doesn't matter what it looks like or what anybody else thinks. So every day I get on the mat and see what I'm feeling. What is my breath like? What is my energy like? Where am I tight? Where am I loose? And who is this "me" anyway, and who's asking—and who cares? All of that goes onto the mat.

DIANA KREBS

I try to do yoga every day for about 30 minutes. I do a couple of Sun Salutations and then whatever my body needs, usually some hip openers (I sit a lot during the

SEANE CORN'S
Home Practice

When Seane does a more organized practice, she breaks it down into six sections–Sun Salutations; standing poses; backbends; forward bends; inversions; and Corpse Pose–moving through the full cycle of life from birth to death.

- ꙮ Begin in Supta Baddha Konasana (Reclining Bound Angle Pose), which epitomizes birth, offering an opportunity for grounding and intention.

- ꙮ Move through several Surya Namaskar (Sun Salutations), experiencing the fluidity of childhood.

- ꙮ Choose a variety of standing poses, which signify ego development in young adulthood, where we learn to stand on our own two feet.

- ꙮ Open into backbends, which exemplify our twenties and thirties, a time of *tapas* (fierce determination) when we are finding our place in the world.

- ꙮ Release into a few forward bends and hip openers, which represent our forties, fifties, and sixties, and help us create time and space for deeper reflection.

- ꙮ Turning upside down in an inversion can help us mix things up and approach the world from a different perspective.

- ꙮ Rest in Savasana (Corpse Pose), which symbolizes transcendence, surrender, and death.

day) and some twists. I love balances and they come easy to me. In my home practice, I have learned that it's not about perfection, but about fun and what my body really needs. For years I was caught up in what I thought should be the perfect alignment. But, the fact is the body is never the same, so I can't expect alignments to be the same. I no longer beat myself up for my basic practice or the fact that, after all these years, I still can't get into Crow Pose.

FELICIA TOMASKO

Avoid the trap of feeling that it is all or nothing—that you must have the perfect space or nothing, the perfect amount of time or nothing. Let yourself practice in spare moments, in whatever space you have available. Create the sacred with intention, with breath, and with the boundary of a mat—or the mind.

I live in a small space, and I share that space with my office, so I have no dedicated place to practice; I must create internal space with what I have. Sometimes I meditate in bed before going to sleep or right when I wake up. During the day, I'll take meditation breaks on my couch, with my dog in my lap. I love to do yoga on my front porch (which is a great, flat, open space), in my backyard, next to my bed on the hardwood floor, or in a corner of the living room. Wherever I can lay down a mat or a cushion becomes sacred space. I allow myself to be flexible with the creation of sacred space, letting go of the need to have rigid rules about what it needs to look like.

❧

Seane Corn does an energizing practice outside of her Southern California yurt, which overlooks the Pacific Ocean.

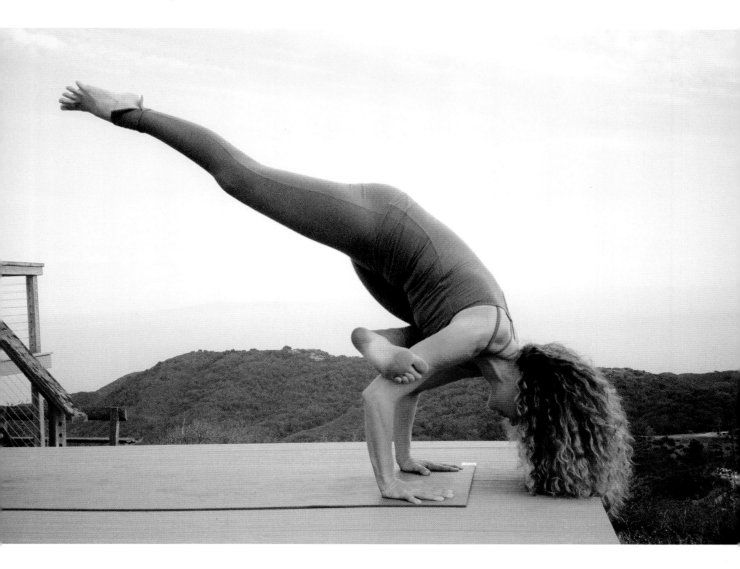

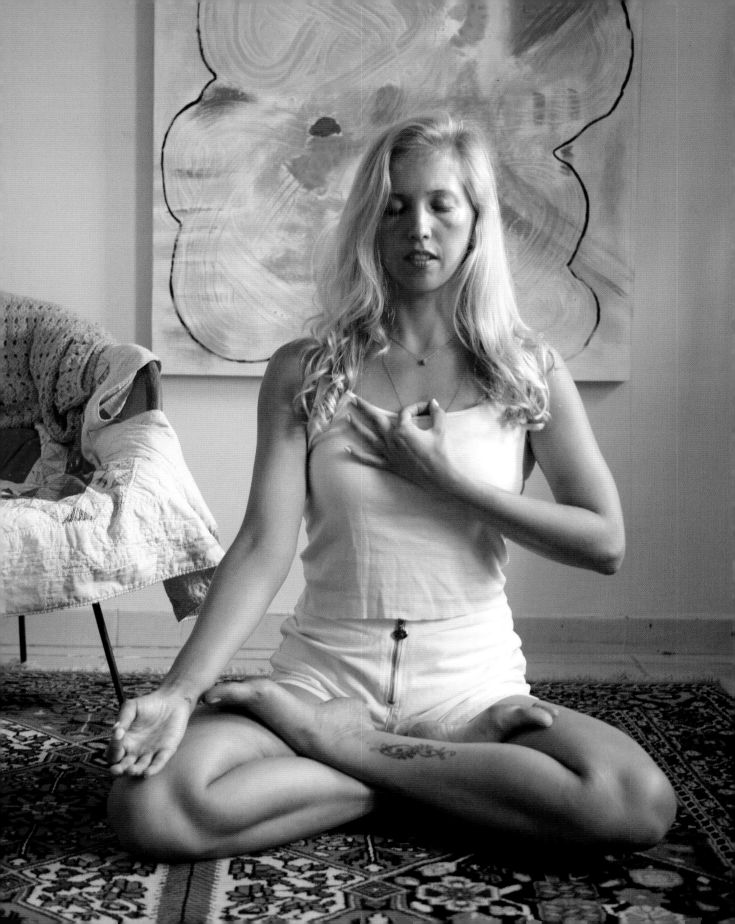

Rolf Sovik's Five Ways to Recharge Your Asana Practice

It's Monday morning and you're ready to begin your asana practice. Unrolling your mat, you listen for the inner voice that guides your movements. But today, that voice is wavering, and your energy is uninspired. How can you breathe new life into your routine?

What follows is a collection of ideas that may restore the spark to your practice if it has lately gone missing, or simply make your practice a bit more engaging. And if these ideas work, then it's likely that as time passes you'll add to them, using your own practice and the challenges of your own body as a guide.

OPTION ONE | Internalize your practice by closing your eyes or softening your gaze as you work. No practice thrives for long without turning inward. Closing your eyes brings a more intensely internal experience to what we do. Sensations that might have been missed are brought to awareness, and those that are normally encountered come to our attention more quickly. Start your practice with a period of breath awareness to relax and anchor this internal focus.

In addition to the sensitivity you gain from closing your eyes, working with your eyes closed can add a surprising challenge to a pose. For example, stretch your assumption about the importance of keeping a fixed gaze in balance poses by closing your eyes the next time you try Tree Pose.

OPTION TWO | Work as if you are healing. Each of us has had an injury that resulted in restricted movement. But then one day we felt that magic sensation of healing, the feeling that we were becoming well again—not completely back to normal, but that muscles were nonetheless beginning to relax, and it felt good to stretch them and explore movements we had not felt in many days or weeks.

Every yoga pose can be performed with this attitude. Stretch, strengthen, and move with the sense that your body is healing from old and forgotten injuries. Monitor the pace of your work so that you do not work faster than the healing process really allows. Don't be swayed into thinking that some other approach will work better. Only healing and increasing vitality merit your energy and enthusiasm.

OPTION THREE | Let poses come to you through longer holding times. If you've become used to moving into and out of poses quickly, you may discover that your habit allows you to avoid feeling the pose. Longer holding times will transform this. But don't dive deeply into a pose and hold it with desperate resolve. Instead, use preparatory movements as a way to explore it, and then hold a version that is safe and pleasantly challenging. Come back to some poses later in your routine in order to move more deeply into them. This will give gravity, your breath, and your inner sensitivity time to let each pose come to you.

OPTION FOUR | Deepen your awareness of muscle tension and resistance. Despite our intention to relax, all of us paradoxically tighten our muscles and resist relaxing at subtle levels. Longer holding times will help us discover these more subtle tensions, but recognizing them also requires increased sensitivity.

OPTION FIVE | Gain a working knowledge of muscles and joints. Without this, it's difficult to analyze the forces at work in any particular pose. Movement takes place when a muscle (or gravity) acts on a joint. We are all familiar, for example, with the experience of hamstring muscles stretched to their limit by a forward bend. But just why does forward bending have this inevitable effect? The answer lies in the location of the attachments of the hamstrings, the action of forward bending on those attachments, the relationship of hamstrings to knee and hip joints, and the nature of forward bending in respect to pelvic and lower back stability. Hit the books if you are uncertain about these anatomical details—it will give you confidence in your understanding of each pose.

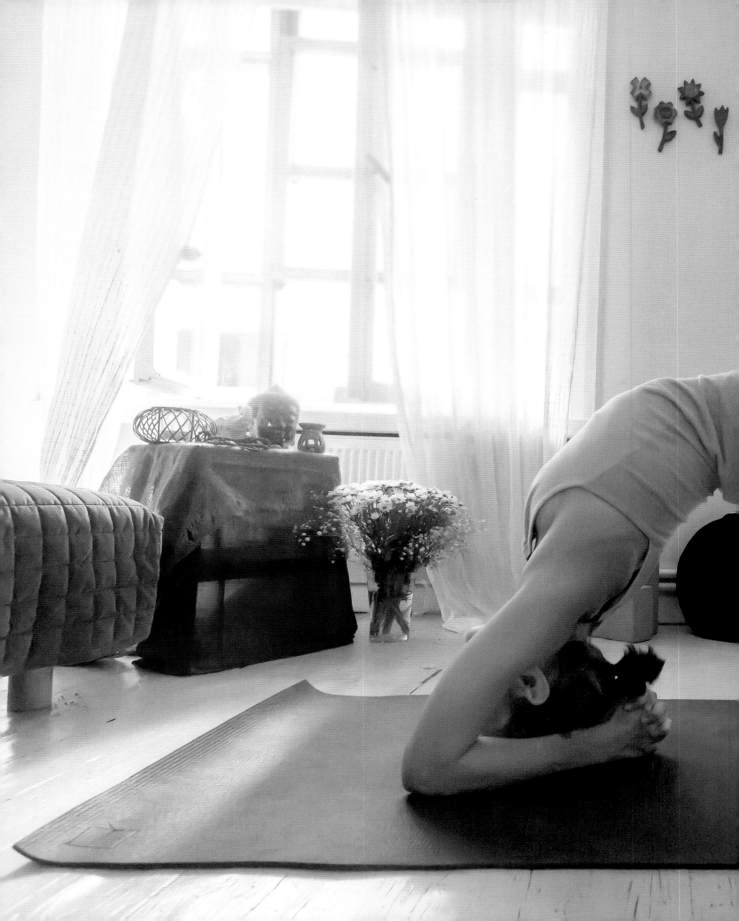

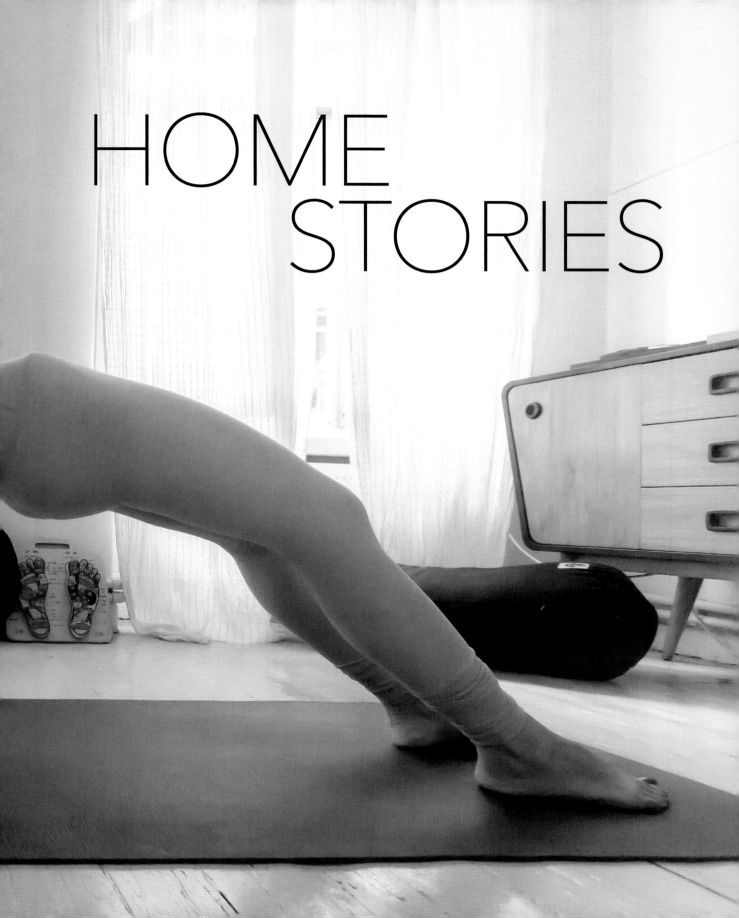

HOME
STORIES

Seane Corn

LOS ANGELES, CALIFORNIA | YOGA TEACHER/ACTIVIST

An internationally celebrated yoga teacher and creator of Off the Mat, Into the World, Seane is known for her activism, unique self-expression, and inspirational style of teaching that incorporates the physical and mystical aspects of yoga.

My practice now is always prayer based, whether I do a 15-minute practice or a 90-minute one. I wake up in the morning and brew a cup of Fortune Delight tea. I quickly scan the news of the day online, noting the current crises being reported. Then I move into my practice room—sometimes I practice in my yurt (which is four miles from my house) and other times I practice at home. Wherever I am, I roll out my mat in front of my altar, light my candles, press my palms together at my heart, and set my intention for my practice. I might have a particular circumstance in mind or a certain person. If I'm focusing on a person, I often put a photo on the altar or something that reminds me of him or her before I pray.

As I begin the asana portion of my practice, every movement, every breath allows me to reflect on what's happening. If it's a person, I'll reflect on what's going on, what he or she needs. If it's a particular event or circumstance, I'll reflect on the specifics—who the leaders are, who the innocents are, what the costs are in terms of lives and society. Every movement I do becomes a physical expression of that prayer, a

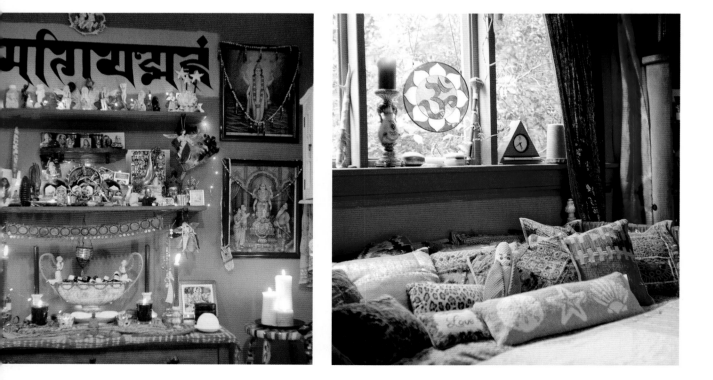

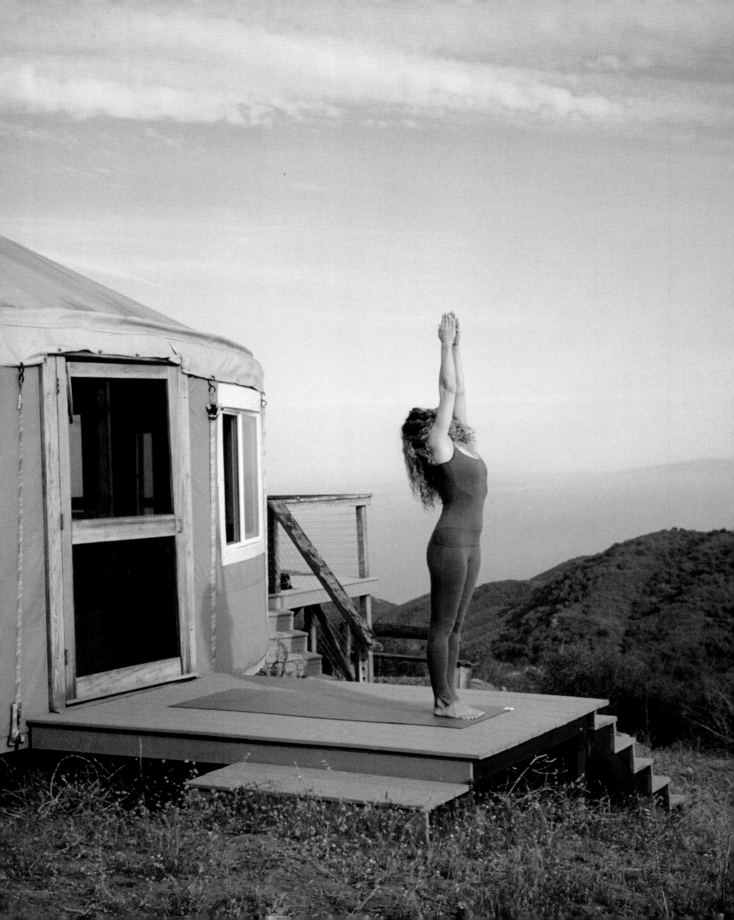

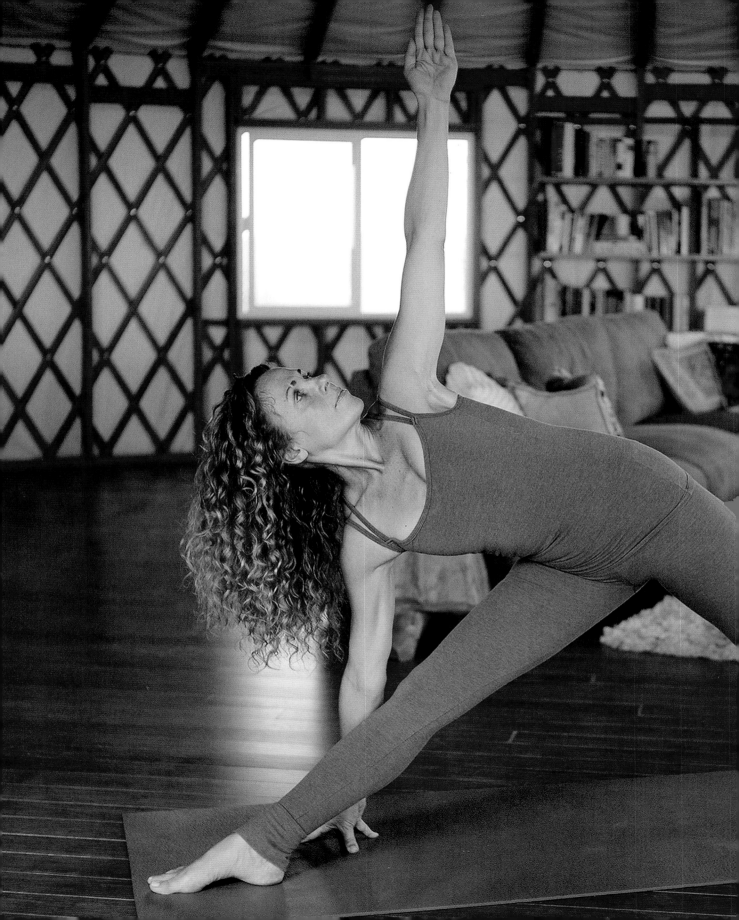

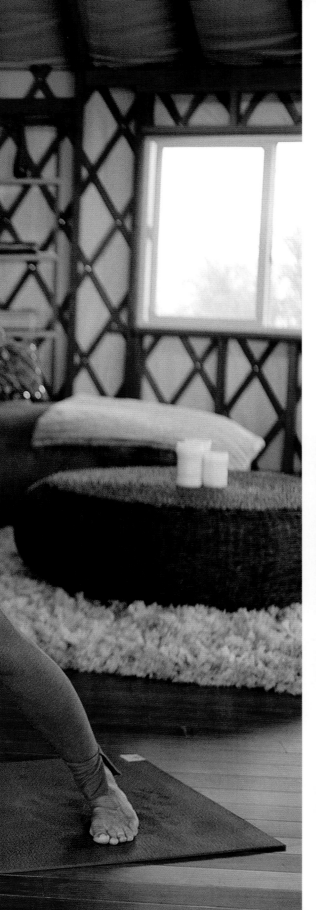

meditation in action; every breath allows me to pull energy in and send energy out, acknowledging the violence, acknowledging the circumstance, acknowledging the pain. Even if I fall out of a pose, that becomes an expression of prayer, too. I often go toward what breaks my heart.

My physical practice is a way for me to release tension so that, at the end of the practice, I can sit, meditate, and be present to the world itself. Making my practice prayer based is the way I can make yoga bigger than myself, more healing. I do yoga in service to altruism. If I've had an intense yang day, regardless of what I *should* do, I'll move into a yin practice. If my day has been mellow, I'll do a more energetic yang practice.

I used to bring all my little statuettes with me when I traveled and set up a little altar, but that became too impractical, going through customs and airport security. So now I take a travel mat with me and maybe sprinkle some essential oils into the carpet in my hotel room before I begin.

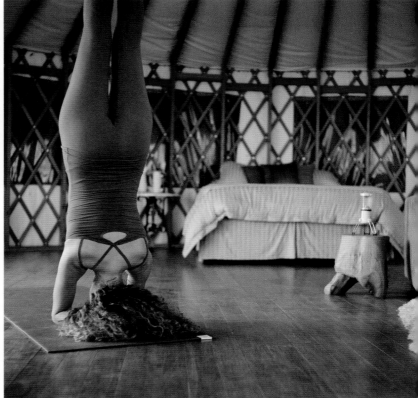

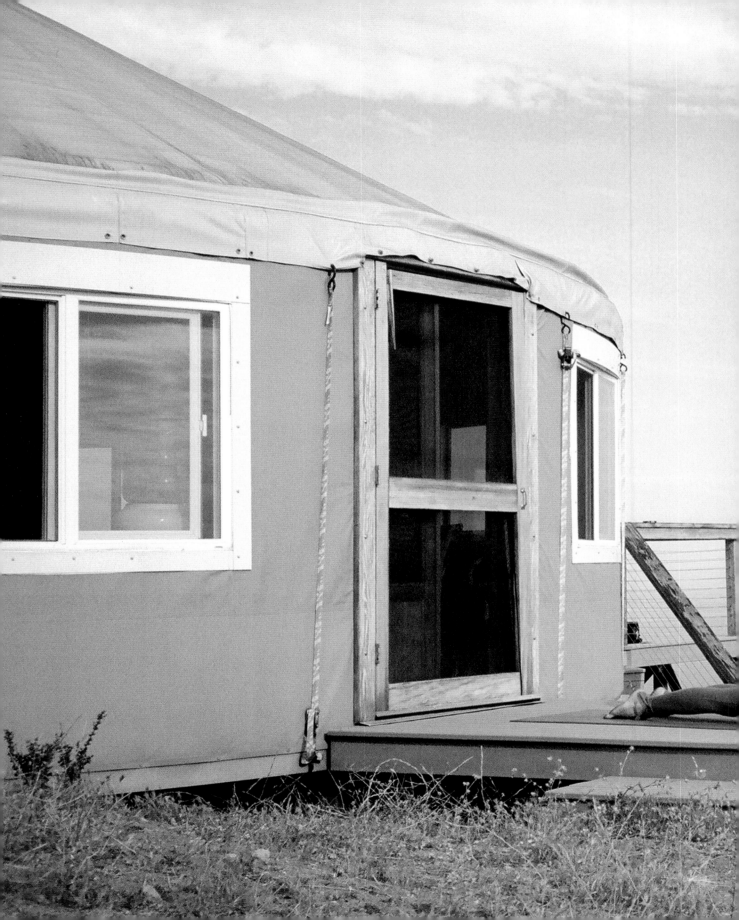

"You cannot practice without love. It's got to have romance in it. It has to turn you on."

Sharon Gannon

NEW YORK & WOODSTOCK, NEW YORK | AUTHOR/YOGA TEACHER/YOGA STUDIO CO-OWNER

A modern Renaissance woman, Sharon is a passionate animal-rights advocate, accomplished musician, artist, and writer. Along with David Life, she created the Jivamukti Yoga lineage, a path to enlightenment through compassion for all beings.

My practice is something I do for God. Period. In my life, I want to live for God and so I have to make that real. I have to toughen up. I have to discipline myself to do things that I might not feel like doing every day to just get over me. (*What do I want to do? What feels good to me?*) After sixty-three years, I don't want to keep that attitude going on. I want to move away from it, at least ease up on it. In bhakti yoga, everything you do you try to think of God before

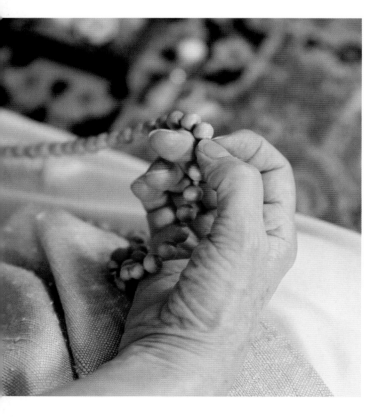

you do it. As soon as I'm conscious of being awake, I've trained myself to remember and talk to God. Make me an instrument of thy will. Allow me to be your servant. Use me today so that I can bring happiness to others; so that I can enhance this world, not just be a selfish taker; so that I can increase your bliss. If God is *sat chit*, mostly *ananda*, I'm into increasing that ananda, God's bliss. That's what I want to do, that's what I'm devoted to doing. I have my own personal way of making my offerings to God every morning.

I do asana in the afternoon. Asana is the way to deal with our karmas. Our bodies are made of our karmas. I have to be comfortable in this body in order to be able to let go of my fascination with me as this mortal personality, this ego being. I have to first of all feel at ease with me. Asanas help us to do that. But the body is a conglomerate of the residue of all of our past relationships. So it's therapy. When I sit in the morning and do my eight rounds of *japa* (mantra) meditation, I don't want to be distracted by thoughts about other people and issues that I am dealing with here or there. So doing a short asana practice, some *kriyas* and pranayama, helps to clear all that out first. And then I can meditate quite directly and keep my mind on God. Why do I do that practice every morning? Because it feels good. When I don't do it, I don't feel good and I don't like to not feel good!

If I'm rushed for time, I do my practice mentally. If I've got to get on an airplane and I've overslept and a car is waiting for me and I haven't done all those *pujas* (offerings to the deity), I'll sit in the back of the cab and I'll do the whole thing in my mind. That's when you know that the practice has borne fruit. You know exactly what comes next. You don't really think

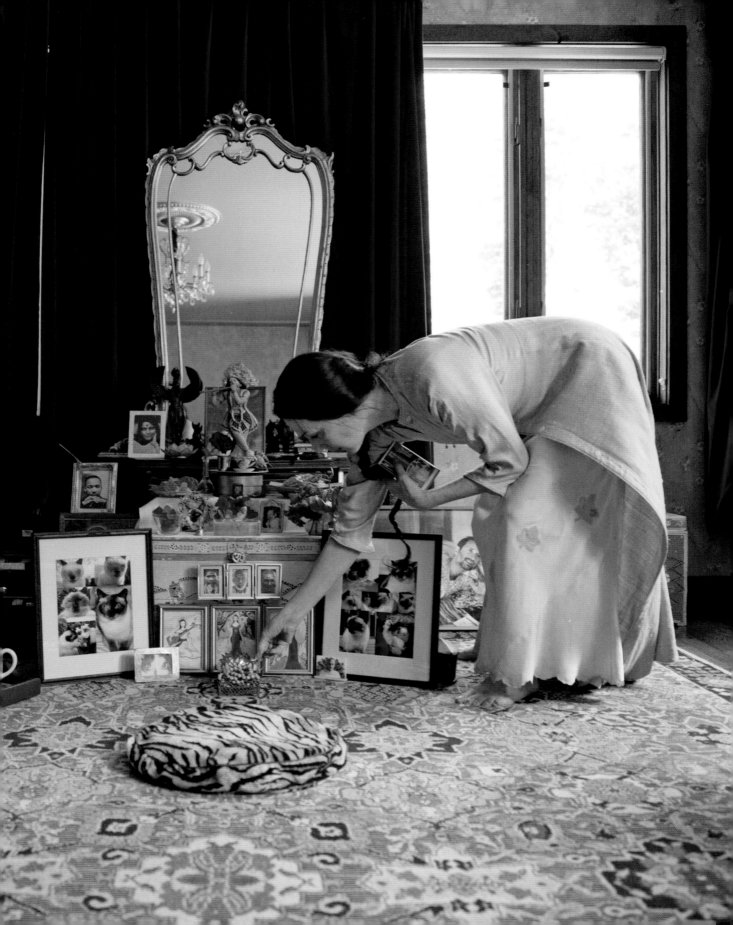

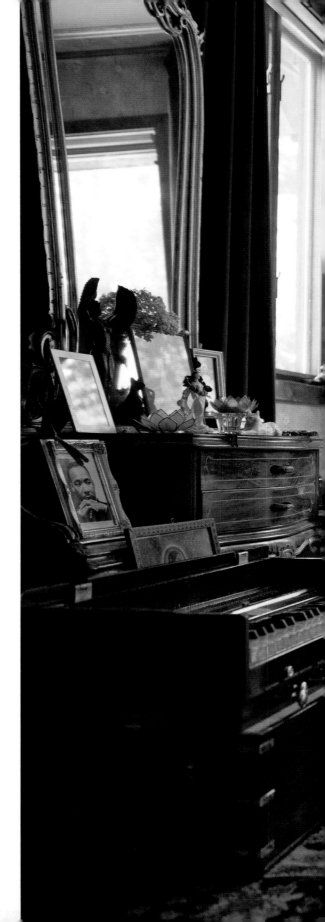

SHARON'S PRACTICE ADVICE

❂ You have to want to practice at home, and you have to want to make the practice part of your life wherever you are. You're not always going to be able to go to your favorite neighborhood yoga studio, so you need to be able to take yoga home with you.

❂ Start small! Meditation is daunting to people when they hear that someone meditates for an hour. *Oh my! Do I have to do that?* No. Just sit, for 1 minute. Close your eyes, let go. Breathe in, breathe out. Do that for a week. Set a timer. And then the next week, do it for 2 minutes. The point is, just do it.

❂ The key word is *doable*. Home practice shouldn't be a huge, goal-oriented thing. Pick something that's within your means.

about it. It's become part of you. OK, I wasn't able to do those eight rounds of japa, so I'll do it walking down the street, in the subway, in a cab. I have found a way to do that. I can do my magic 10 asana sequence (see page 216) in about 7 minutes! You can find time.

You cannot practice without love. It's got to have love in it, romance in it. It has to turn you on. It would be stale and boring to me if I were doing it only for myself. I'm doing it for God, for my teachers; the prayers in the practice are integrated with the names of my teachers. There's magic in the name, in God's name. When I say the names of my teachers, they are instantly with me and suddenly I'm not just me by myself doing a routine. I'm checking in with those other beings. All the love that I have is rekindled, every single day. From other worlds. Simultaneously.

I do a full 90-minute asana practice in the afternoon and I always, always do it with music. The sequence that I do, and have been doing for years, doesn't vary. Sometimes I'll spend a longer time in some poses on some days, and other poses on other days, but it's basically the same.

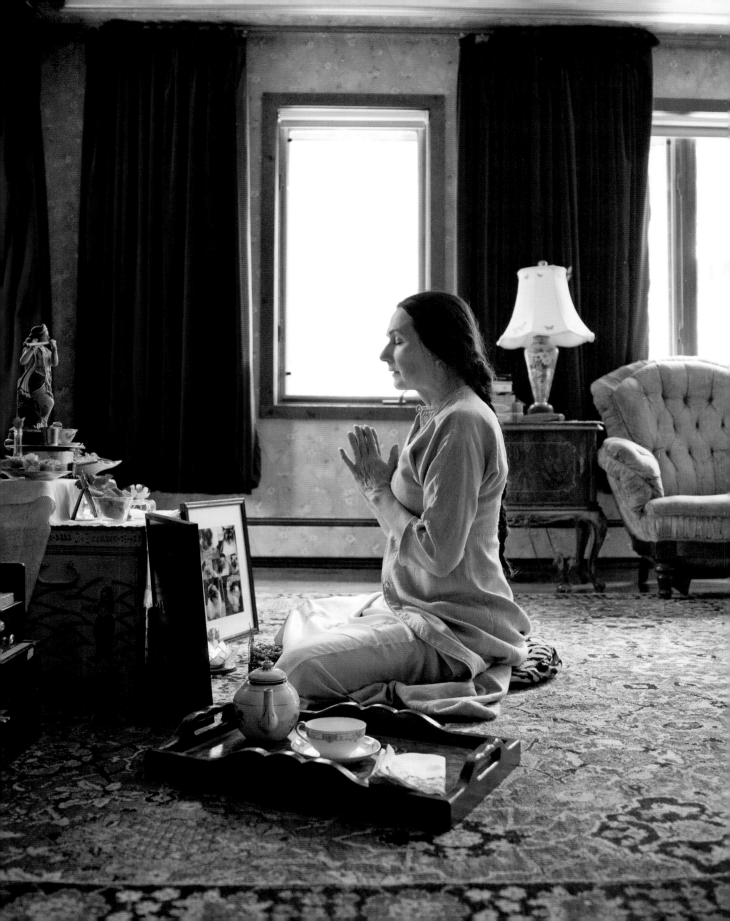

"Home practice arises spontaneously out of a need to do the best you can do in life."

David Life

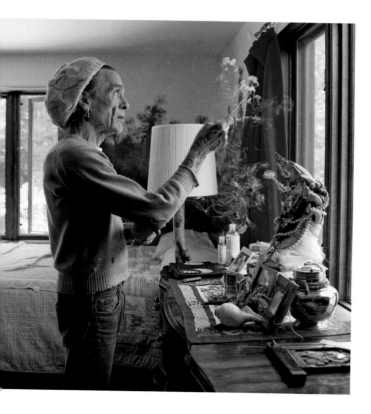

NEW YORK & WOODSTOCK, NEW YORK | YOGA TEACHER/YOGA STUDIO CO-OWNER

As cofounder of Jivamukti Yoga, David has helped bring the ancient teachings alive, making them relevant to the contemporary world, with the blessing of his gurus Nirmalananda, Pattabhi Jois, and Sri Brahmananda Sarasvati.

For a home practice to work, you need a fully functional tool kit so you're not at a loss for what to do. You also need to be told specifically what to do by a guru or by your teachers. What we're talking about here is "home practice," something that's totally self-originated and not enforced by outside regimens or anything else. Home practice arises spontaneously out of a need or a desire to fulfill the expectations of your teachers, to do the best you can do in life. There's no program to make you do that—it's all up to you.

DAVID'S PRACTICE ADVICE

🌱 The ancient yogis were wanderers; they had no permanent home. So they would have to get up in the morning, get moving, find or beg for their food, prepare it, find another camp, establish another place to sleep, and *then* practice yoga! But when you have a home, you get to stay put and take many of those things out of the equation. You don't have to move on and beg for food, so you have that time to practice. You don't have to worry about where you're going to sleep tomorrow night, so you can use that time for yoga.

🌱 If you can keep any distractions to a minimum—by avoiding television and unplugging the Internet and phones at night—you can free up a big chunk of time for your yoga practice.

I have a schedule sort of similar to Sharon's. I spend some portion of my day doing things around here—administrative duties, chores, repairs, cleaning. But my mornings are dedicated to spiritual practice. I try to keep my practice integrated into the rest of my day. I'll often stop and write notes to myself when I'm on my mat, notes that aren't necessarily asana based. Something interesting on the radio may catch my attention (I listen to the radio all the time—alternative, radio talk shows, music), so I'll stop, jot something

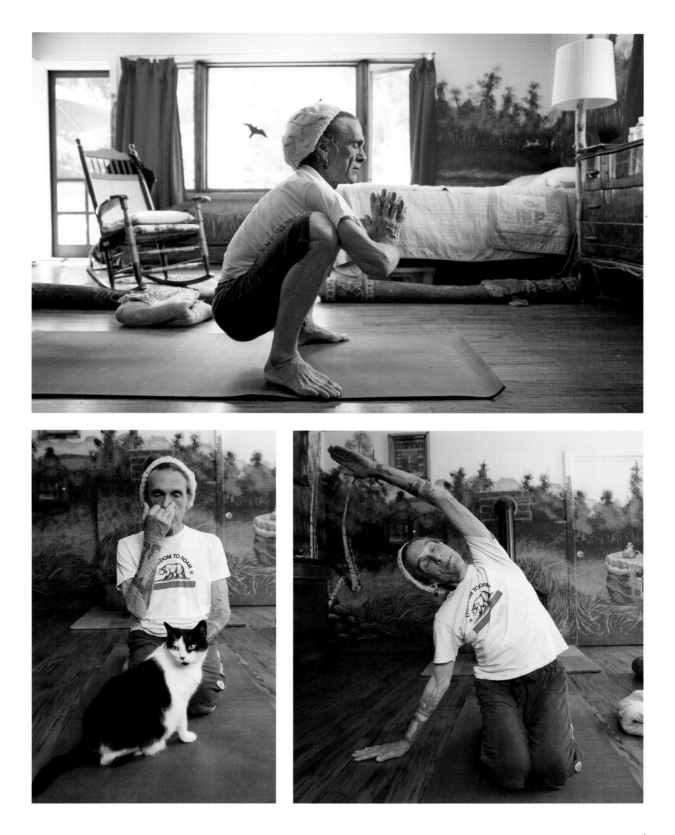

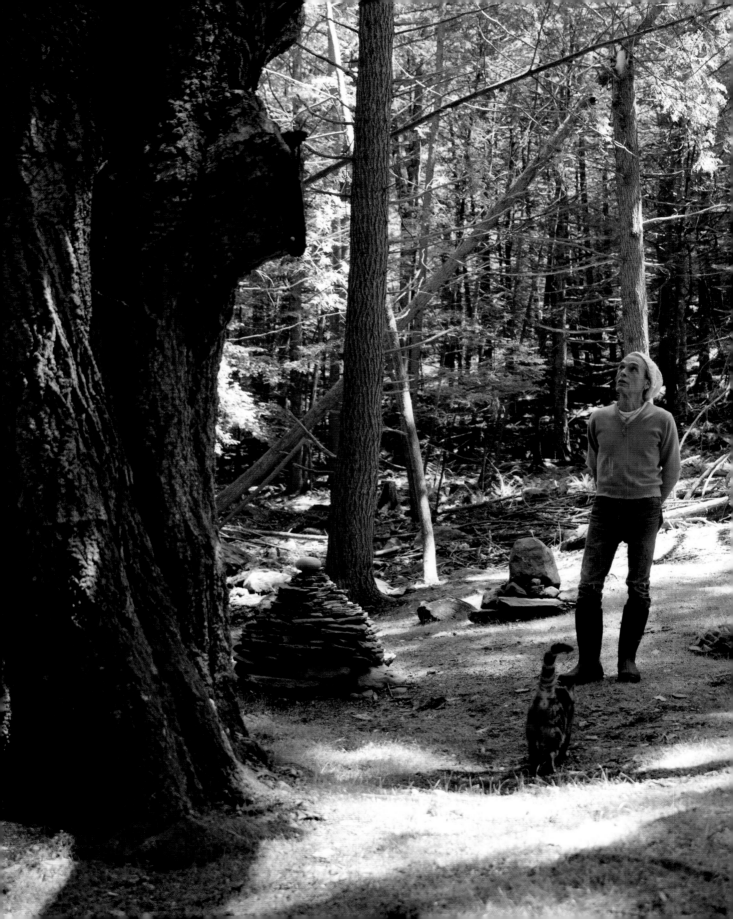

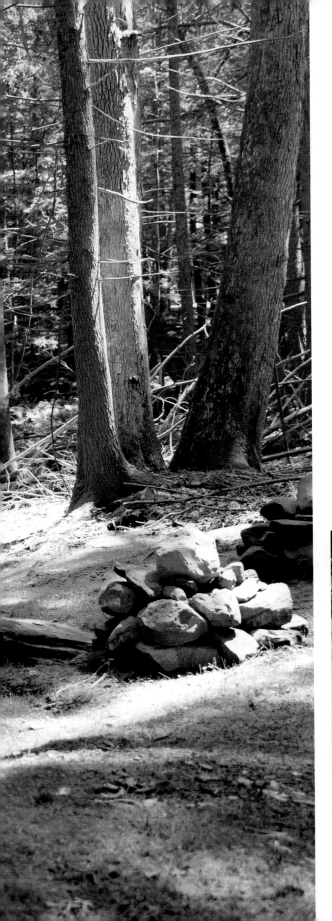

down, and revisit it later. Our cats of course can be a big distraction—they climb on top, burrow underneath, and make it hard to move!

The first thing I do when I get up is make coffee. And then I clean the cat box and make the cats breakfast so they have a morning meal. I make poached eggs for them or oatmeal—that's how I feed them. To me, that's *seva* (service), a purifying gift, because all these cats are rescue cats and I am able to care for them. In the same vein, I then feed the animals that visit our land—the birds, turkeys, deer, bears, foxes, squirrels, and chipmunks.

There's a ritualistic aspect to everything I do, and feeding the animals is really no different. Once that is done, I perform several more offerings. Outside, I recite mantras as I bathe and care for the Shiva lingam. Often I'll walk to Grandmother Oak and ask for her blessing. Inside, I do house-blessing rituals with mantra; *pujas* (offerings) and mantra to my gurus; and then I practice pranayama, asana, and meditation.

Like Sharon, if I have to rush to catch a bus or drive into the city, I can do my pujas in my mind and that feels just fine to me. I do the same asana sequence every day; every day I give the lingam a bath and repeat my mantras in the same way so I can just close my eyes and see the whole thing unfolding.

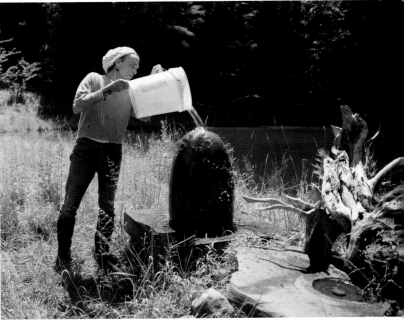

"My room is a private and personal refuge and very much a designated sacred space."

Nicki Doane

MAUI, HAWAII | YOGA TEACHER/YOGA STUDIO OWNER

Combining asana, pranayama, meditation, philosophy, and poetry, Nicki creates a yoga "life-support system" that can be carried into daily life. Her teacher Pattabhi Jois said to her, "You, yoga, many lifetimes," and that says it all.

We built our main house eight years ago and it's significantly bigger than our old little cabin. In the new house I have a special yoga room all to myself, upstairs off my bedroom. I have to walk through the closet to get to it. It has high windows and gorgeous Tibetan red plastered walls. Originally, I wanted it to be more of a cell with no windows at all, but I relented. I love practicing there because I can get out of bed and be in the yoga room in seconds.

My room is a private and personal refuge and very much a designated sacred space for my practice. It has an altar with many photographs and special things

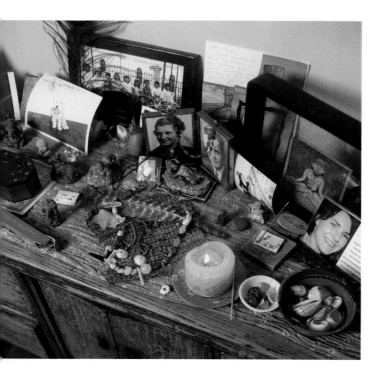

NICKI'S PRACTICE ADVICE

🖐 Creating a home practice is more difficult than you think, but it will help you get to know and care for yourself better. Start by designating a space in your home just for your practice—it could be a corner of a room or a shaded deck, or anywhere you can leave your mat unrolled and your props out, and even put up a small altar.

🖐 Home practice should start slowly and build gradually. It might be only 10 minutes at the beginning, but it will gradually lengthen.

🖐 Pick three poses that are personally significant for you right now. Only pick three. I'm not talking about three of your favorite poses, but three that will challenge you. Work on those poses four to six times for a week. Start to figure out which additional poses will help you get into your three personal poses.

that I have collected throughout my entire life. I am blessed that it is tucked into a little nook of our house that most people never even see. When I need to think or process or cry, I head to my yoga room, where I feel safe to be who I am and feel whatever I feel.

There are some days I literally drag myself to the mat and just lie there in Savasana and that's my practice. I have practiced for so long that I have a cellular

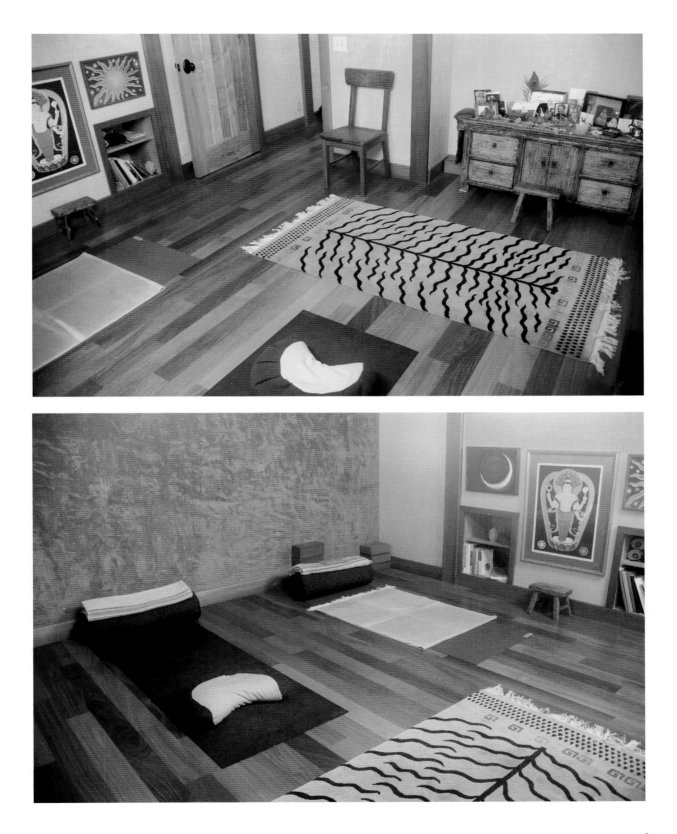

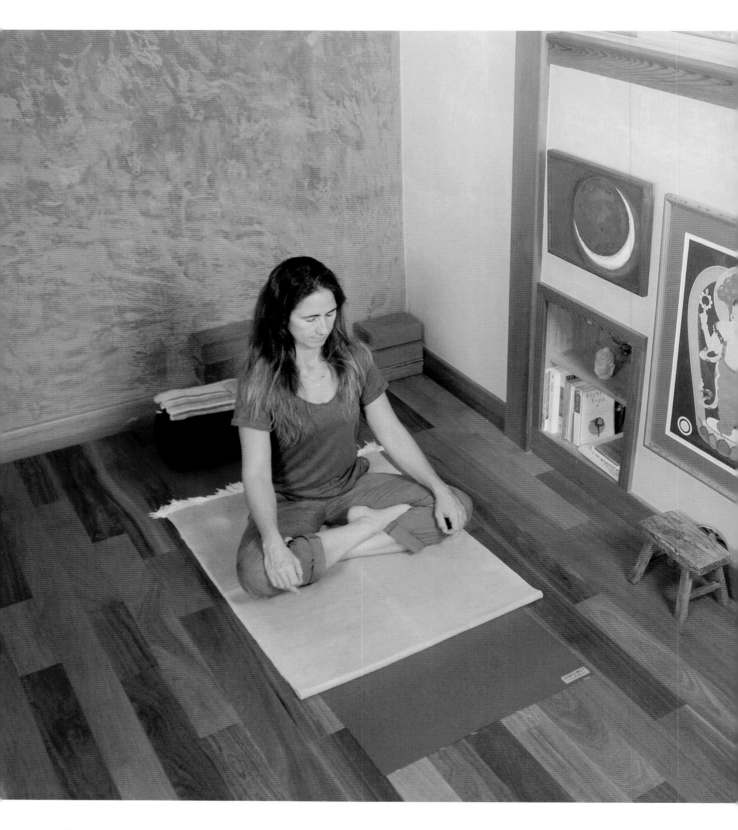

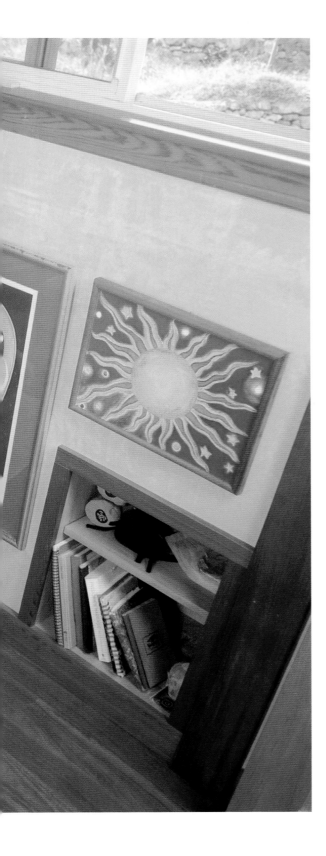

NICKI'S SAMPLE PRACTICE

- Sit in a simple cross-legged position
- Nadi Shodhana Pranayama (Alternate Nostril Breathing) for 3 to 5 minutes
- Uttanasana (Standing Forward Bend) for 1 minute
- Adho Mukha Svanasana (Downward-Facing Dog) for 2 to 3 minutes
- Balasana (Child's Pose) for 1 minute
- Surya Namaskar A (Sun Salutation A) three times
- Trikonasana (Triangle Pose) for 1 minute on each side
- Virabhadrasana II (Warrior II) for 30 seconds on each side
- Setu Bandha Sarvangasana (Supported Bridge Pose) two times from the floor
- Apanasana (Knees-to-Chest Pose)
- Ardha Jathara Parivartanasana (Supine Belly Twist with Bent Knees)
- Savasana (Corpse Pose)

memory of how it feels to do yoga and I know that if I don't do it I will only feel worse.

Over the years, when I had to practice in the living room or in my bedroom, it was difficult to stay focused on me and my mat. I would find myself looking at all the dust under the bed or under the couch and wanting to clean it up right then and there; or the phone would ring; or any number of mundane household chores would be more in the front of my consciousness. Now, my practice space is so wonderful and so removed from the rest of the house that it feels sacred, and everything that I do in that room relates to yoga completely.

When I first started yoga it was all about the poses. But, as my practice has grown and matured, it has moved to a deeper, subtler level. I find the chanting of the sutras very inspiring and I often begin each day with that.

"We all need a place where we can sit down and listen. That's what home practice can bring."

Sarah Powers

SAN FRANCISCO, CALIFORNIA & NEW YORK, NEW YORK | YOGA TEACHER/AUTHOR

As cofounder of the Insight Yoga Institute and author of *Insight Yoga*, Sarah weaves yin and yang yoga, Buddhism, Taoism, and Transpersonal Psychology into an integral practice to discover and enliven the body, heart, and mind.

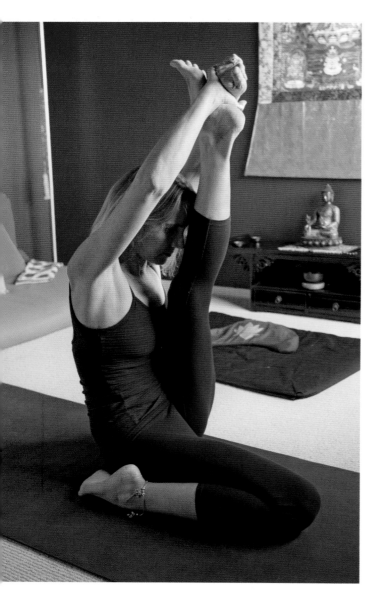

Practicing yoga gives us an opportunity to live with increased integration, to gather together the various parts of our body and mind inside of ourselves so that we can share the whole of our being with the world.

Personal practice calls us to bring something to the mat each time we practice: a sense of curiosity, nonjudgmental interest, and appropriate use of the methods we can tolerate today. We all need a place where we can sit down and listen. And we also need a place where we can move, strengthen, and enjoy our physicality—be demonstrative and not pressured by anyone else's business or judgments. That's what home practice can bring. There's something about having my own dialogue with myself and the universe—and not unfolding someone else in the space—that gives me the freedom to explore and the permission to adjust when something's not working.

We are too often guided by our habits to avoid this or procrastinate that. But during my practice, I can hold myself open to the possibility of being more conscious and more awake. I may have a lot of compulsions and addictions, but not for those moments on my mat. I'm living for my mature self. I can do that. And maybe I can even do that off the mat. The more we do yoga, the more we can reinforce these practices throughout the day, becoming more conscious and more awake.

So much daily activity is time bound. Even in our yoga practice we're not doing enough, not getting far enough and fast enough. Yin is about stillness. If I just do two or three poses, I feel a sense of calm abiding within myself, no matter how anxious or pressured I felt when I began. In this moment, I can experience a breath of fresh air. I can listen and simply *be* rather than focusing on a specific agenda or result.

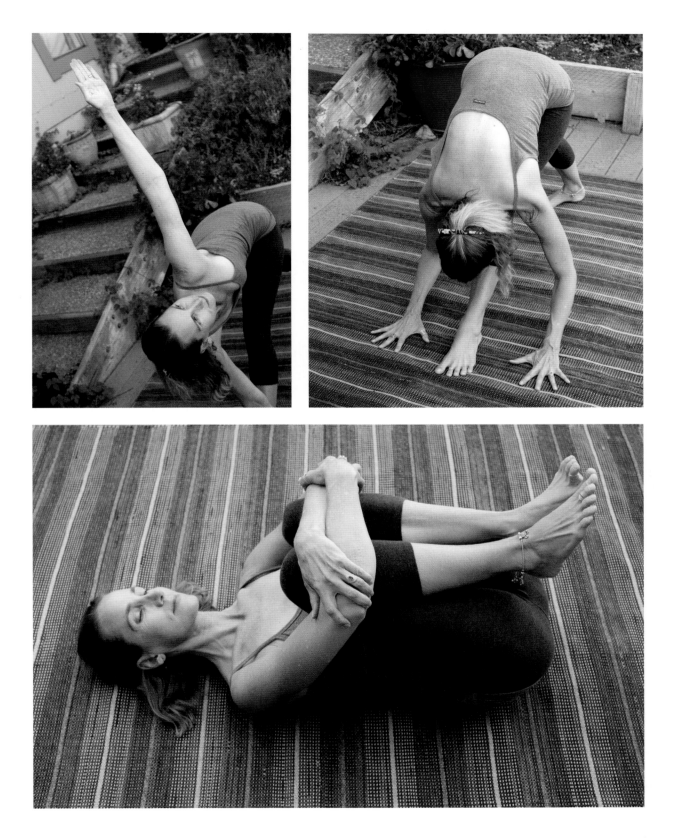

SARAH'S PRACTICE ADVICE

- Borrow insights from your teachers. They've worked with, wrestled, adopted, and adapted yoga for their personal journey. That will give you a template to begin with, and then you can adapt and adjust for the seasons of your own life and make the practice your own.

- Regardless of what you do, always have a beginning, middle, and end to your practice. The beginning should be some kind of check in and grounding; the ending should always include Savasana.

- Do a little bit each day and cultivate a generosity of inquiry. The question, "What do I really need and want?" is more important than, "What is expected of me?"

- Be more inclusive toward the various dimensions of your being—the tightness, the developmental difficulties, the sense of not being worthy.

- Cultivate discipline. Discipline breeds familiarity and brings you to a place where you can recognize yourself. *Oh, yes, it's you again; I know that pattern in my bones.* Familiarize yourself with yourself. Continuity of connection becomes common ground.

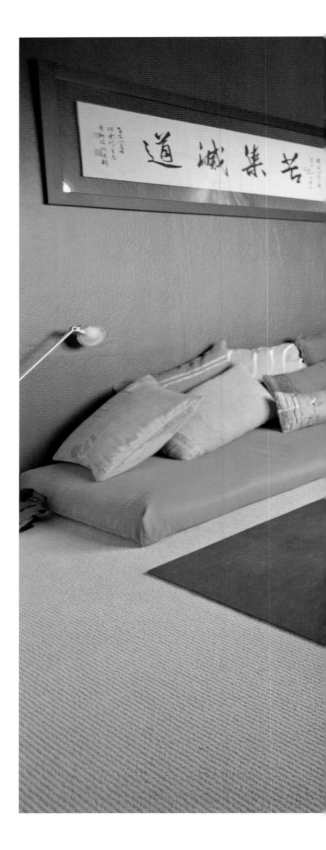

That said, my home practice has become an integration of both aspects—the receptive (yin) and the dynamic (yang). I practice yin because it gives me the ability to slow down and interpret inner cues from inner realms. And then, with yin as my center of gravity, I move into a slower, more deliberate, and juicier yang (vinyasa) practice. Starting with yin reduces any agony of performance I might feel in an active practice. My capacity to relax striving and to invite exploring becomes joyous. Joy can then drive my practice instead of the dryness of discipline. I like to bring a yin attitude inside my yang practice. If I don't set that dial, the pressure to constantly produce, to move, to get stronger causes a lot of stress and problems.

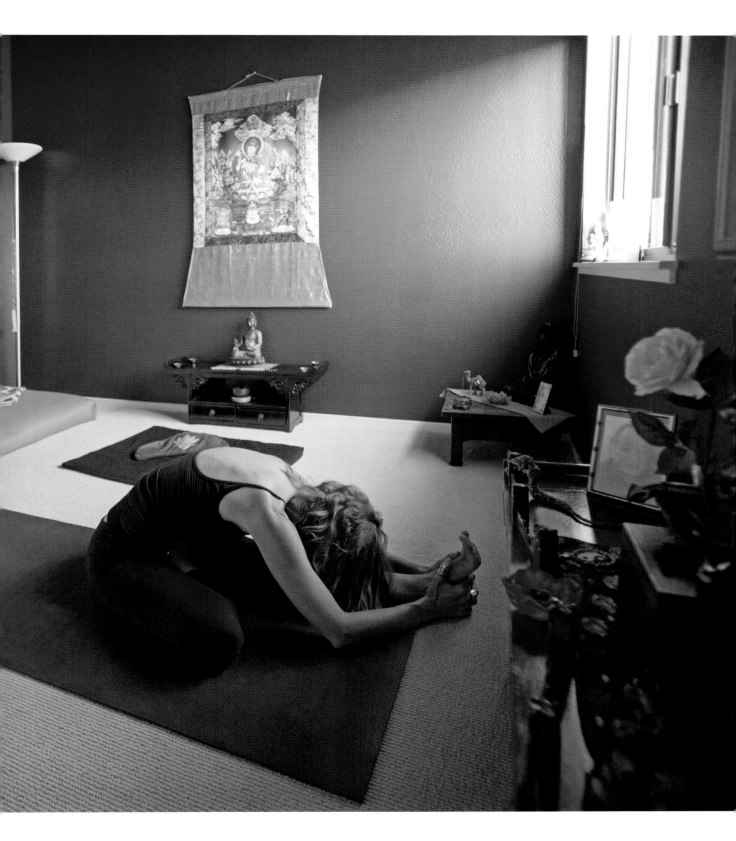

"Practicing alone gives me the opportunity to explore who I am on an intimate level."

Faith Hunter

NEW YORK, NEW YORK & WASHINGTON, DC | YOGA TEACHER

The creator of Spiritually Fly, Faith celebrates every moment of life and uses chanting and music, breath, and movement as a way to encourage students to embrace their unique flow in life—on and off the mat.

When I practice at home, I truly listen and honor where I am emotionally and physically. Some days my practice is restorative and healing, and other days it is a more fluid, high-energy experience.

The practice of yoga has provided and continues to provide comfort, balance, and steadiness during challenging moments. I always know my practice is there, holding a space for my heart. When I do feel challenged, I typically start with a short meditation that I do in bed when I first wake up. It gets me going and provides focus when those uncomfortable thoughts creep in. The meditation includes a little visualization and ends with giving thanks. This approach sets the tone for my day, and inspires my body to move.

I recently returned to New York City. My current home is a cute junior one-bedroom apartment that is also my home office. My space is very personalized. I have an altar with family photos, flowers, pillows, yoga props, mats, lots of books, and other memorable items I've collected over the years. I'm also inspired by my two adorable shih tzus, Yoshi and Sebastian, moving around the apartment. I love watching them shape-shift into Upward-Facing and Downward-Facing Dog.

Practicing alone gives me the opportunity to explore who I am on an intimate level, the time to dive deeper into my mediation practice, and the freedom to move in a way that feels natural to me.

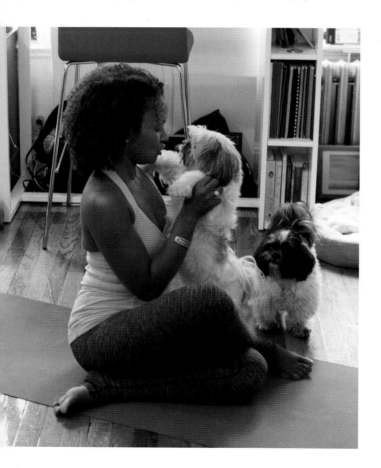

FAITH'S PRACTICE ADVICE

ꕥ Start simple. Don't overwhelm yourself with long practices and complicated sequences. Select a practice time that fits your lifestyle. If you are not a morning person, don't practice at 6:00 a.m.

ꕥ Create a dedicated space, and place items in your space that inspire you.

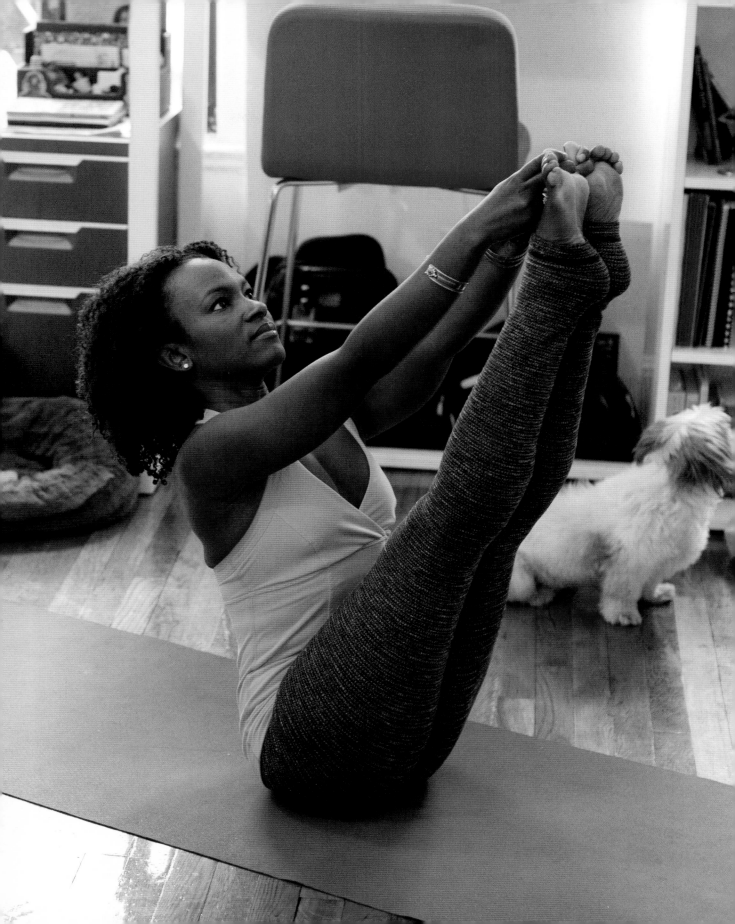

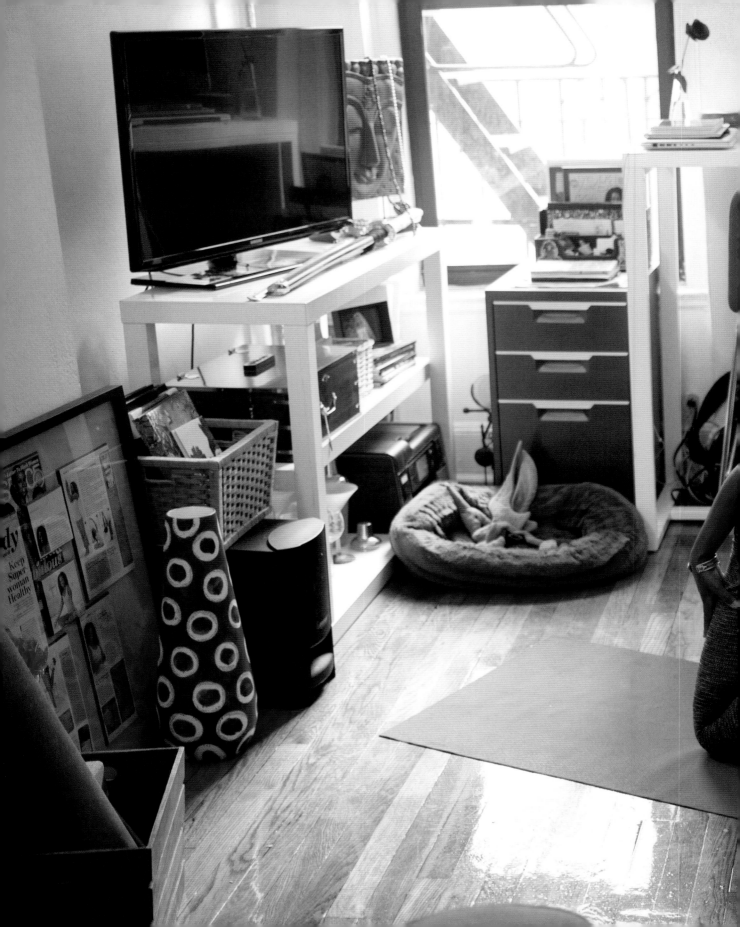

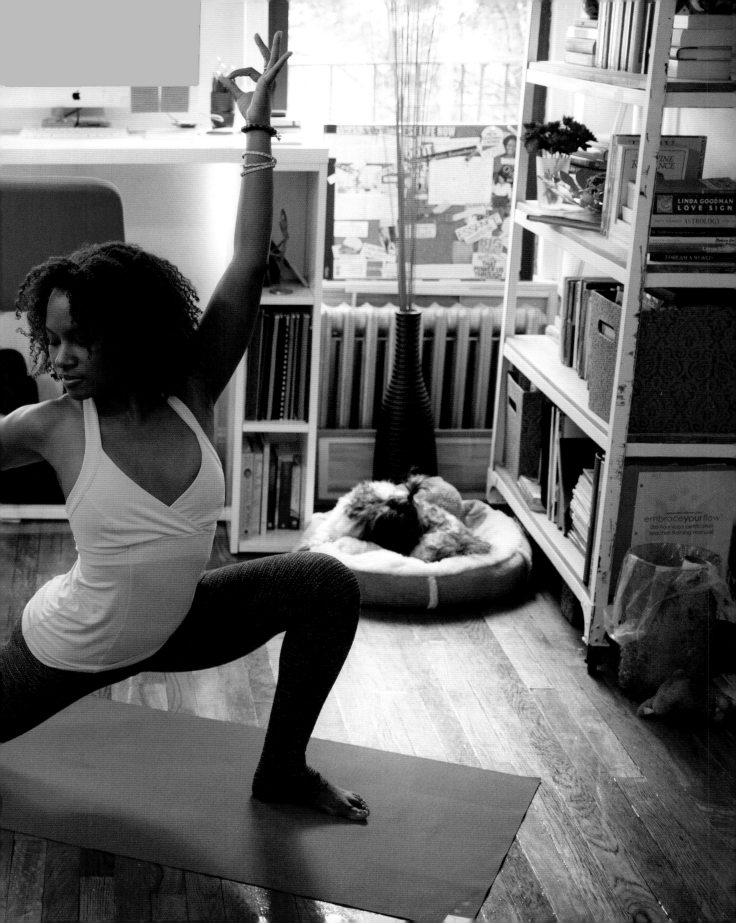

"I do yoga because it calms me enough to think clearly through crises."

Frances Gulland

MARIN COUNTY, CALIFORNIA | SENIOR SCIENTIST

In addition to providing medical care for thousands of seals and sea lions at the Marine Mammal Center in Sausalito, Frances serves as a commissioner for the U.S. Marine Mammal Commission. No wonder she relishes her Power Yoga time.

In our tiny house, all I need for my practice is a quiet space and about two feet around the mat itself. If no one needs it in the morning, I'll use the back study; if the weather cooperates, I'll go outside on the lawn; and in the early evening, when the dining-room area catches the setting sun, I'll set up my mat there.

I do yoga because it calms me enough to think clearly through crises. And because I can dedicate my practice to someone in need that day. Knowing that I'll feel calmer and more relaxed afterward keeps me coming back even as household chores can sometimes make practice difficult to prioritize.

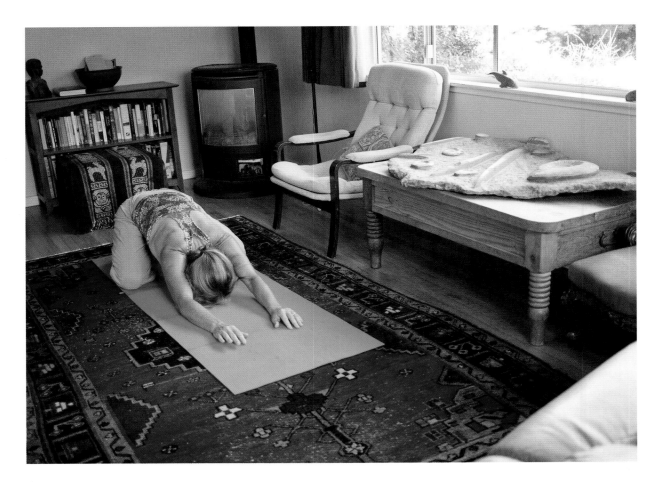

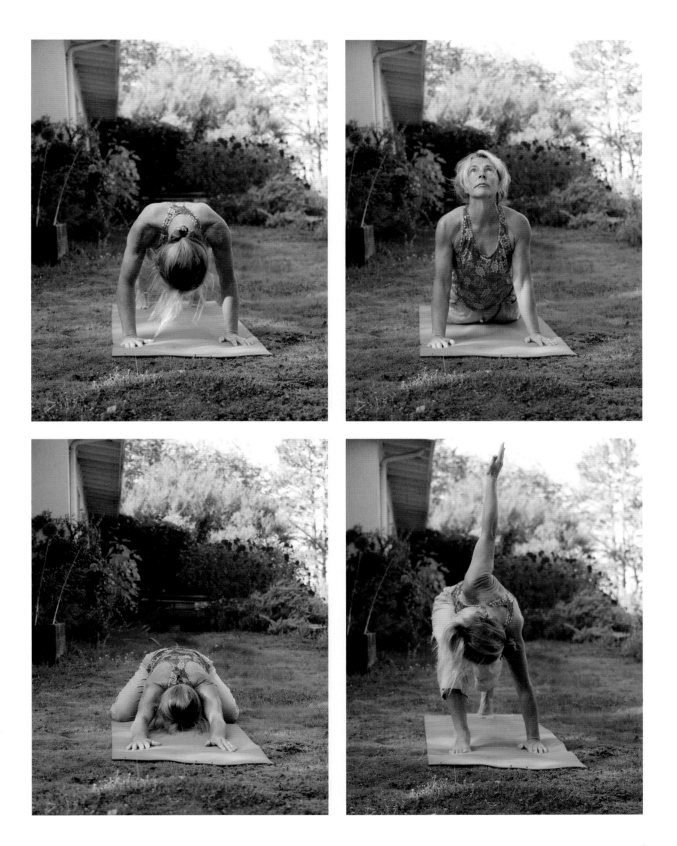

> *"The right moment is this moment and the best place to start is wherever you are."*

Sinem Er

ISTANBUL, TURKEY | YOGA TEACHER

Seamlessly weaving meditation and yoga asana into her practice and her teaching, Sinem credits yoga with healing her body and maintaining her connection to self. Sinem's influences include her teacher Cyndi Lee, founder of OM Yoga.

I live in a small apartment, so my practice space is in my living room. I have a small corner altar and I like to keep it surrounded with fresh flowers—although my cat eats them!—and some candles. I use an oil diffuser to keep the air fresh and smelling nice. I always keep the area clean, and cleaning the area is also part of my little ritual.

When I feel like I lose my center or hope, meditation is my ally. When I've been injured, specific asana

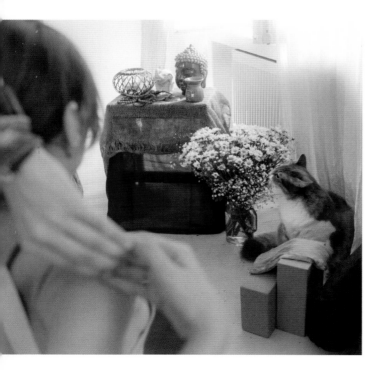

combinations are of great help. For instance, last year I fell down the stairs and broke my coccyx. At first, it was impossible to even take a step, let alone bend in half or go into Downward-Facing Dog. But with the help of props, a lot of deep listening, and doing only upper-body movements, I gradually started to increase my range of motion to Half Sun Salutations, and then I figured out ways to modify my practice to my limitation at that moment. I created a sequence for myself and practiced it every day. I healed so fast that my doctor was in shock. But besides this physical benefit, sticking to the practice itself was my savior, because it helped me maintain the connection to myself, to keep going, despite the hard situation, without losing heart.

My cat Miou came to my life six years ago, when she was only three weeks old. At that time I was working at an advertising agency, and one day I found her in a box, abandoned at my doorstep. I took her in and started to take care of her. Ever since, we have been together and she especially loves being around when I am practicing or teaching at home. She loves sitting on my lap while meditating (she does her own "catitation," I guess), and she enjoys mantras very much. Her presence truly enriches my life and practice and I learn so much from her. I feel truly blessed to have her in my life.

Anything you do can be a way to connect to yourself, as long as you do it with mindfulness. For instance, I don't do a physical practice on moon days or during menstrual cycles; instead, I paint mandalas or read a dharma book or do mantra or chakra meditations.

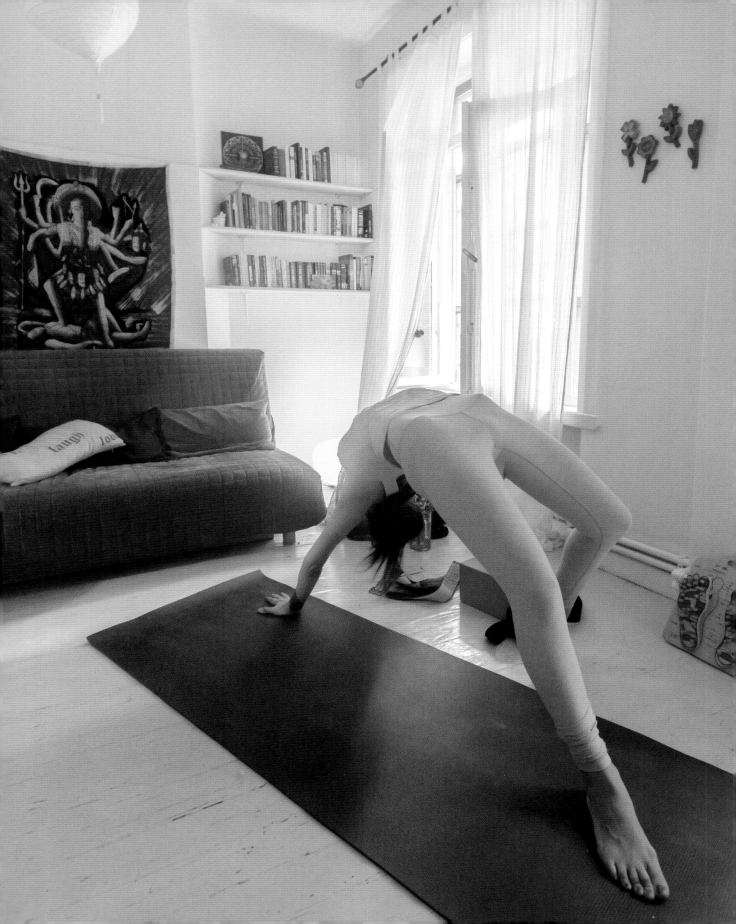

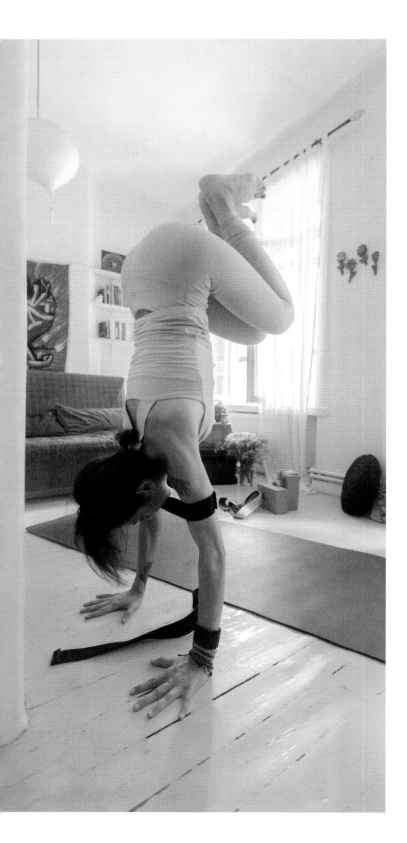

SINEM'S PRACTICE ADVICE

ᵞ One thing to always remember: the right moment is this moment and the best place to start is wherever you are. Begin a personal practice as soon as you take your first class, even if it's only for 10 minutes a day. That will give you access to the most important teacher: the practice itself. Going from class participant to yogi with a personal practice may be one of the most transformative things ever.

ᵞ Make sure you create a space where you won't be disturbed during your personal time. Turn off your phone! Then, ask yourself, what do you really need from your practice at that very moment?

ᵞ Start off with a modest goal: for example, 10 minutes of Sun Salutations in the morning, or 10 minutes breathing deeply in Child's Pose. Take your time to build your own confidence and your own commitment to the idea. Like all habits, it's much easier to do this slowly. When you feel ready, you can expand your sessions.

ᵞ Don't be afraid of messing up or "doing it wrong." Let yourself be vulnerable so you are able to grow. Your practice is your personal time and you must let yourself fall over, dance, move in various ways that feel good, and do whatever works for you. Your yoga practice doesn't have to look like anyone else's yoga practice.

ᵞ If you don't feel very confident about asana combinations, you can always practice with DVDs or online classes.

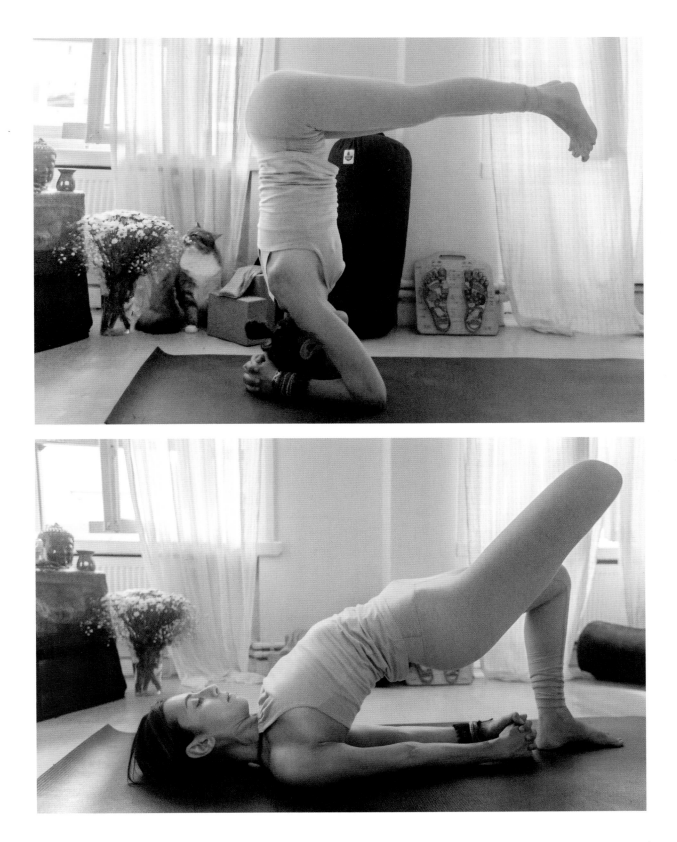

> *"I try to balance the usefulness of my practice and the sacredness of the yoga tradition."*

Annette Söhnlein

BERLIN, GERMANY | YOGA TEACHER

An Anusara-inspired, hatha yoga teacher, Annette infuses her daily yoga and meditation practice with plenty of *bhakti* (love and devotion), which gives her the patience and the power to juggle work and motherhood.

I am a lazy person. Even though I know I need my regular yoga, it takes a lot of effort for me to go on my mat. But there is one thing that gets me there: *bhakti*. Absolute love for what I do is the fire that moves me: if I give myself totally into the yoga, even for a short time each day, I feel the love in and around me. This is what makes my actions in the world better and the yoga is no longer divided from the rest of my life. I know that I am a friendlier person to myself and to others.

I do a short practice in the morning and a wind-down or meditation in the evening every day. After that, I am flexible. Depending on my schedule and the weather, I practice when my body is not too tight from the night and my head is not too loud or busy after working at the computer.

ANNETTE'S PRACTICE ADVICE

- See your yoga practice as your self-healing gift, a gift that you can give yourself every day, any time of the day, every moment it is needed.

- If you are uninspired, read a poem or listen to your favorite music and see if it moves you to your mat. Always practice with a smile.

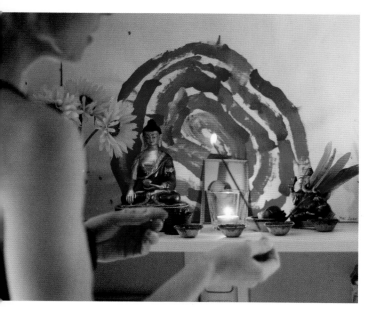

Since my children accept that I am a better and more patient mom after I've done yoga, they accept my time on the mat and sometimes practice their yoga with me, which means crawling under my Downward-Facing Dog, challenging me with the weight of their bodies on my back in Plank Pose, and things like that.

I try to create a balance between the usefulness of my practice and the sacredness of the yoga tradition. Honoring the sacred aspects means I practice when the night kisses the day, the day kisses the night. In these short moments, I make no compromises and take it as a holy time for me and something bigger. In between, I use my practice for what I need: energizing or calming, yin or yang.

There are always Sun Salutations to warm up my body before I do what I need. This doesn't mean that I do only what I would love to do . . . I listen really carefully. *Do I need to ground or do I need to energize? Is there a stiff part in my body that asks for extra love?* I change my asanas every day, just as circumstances

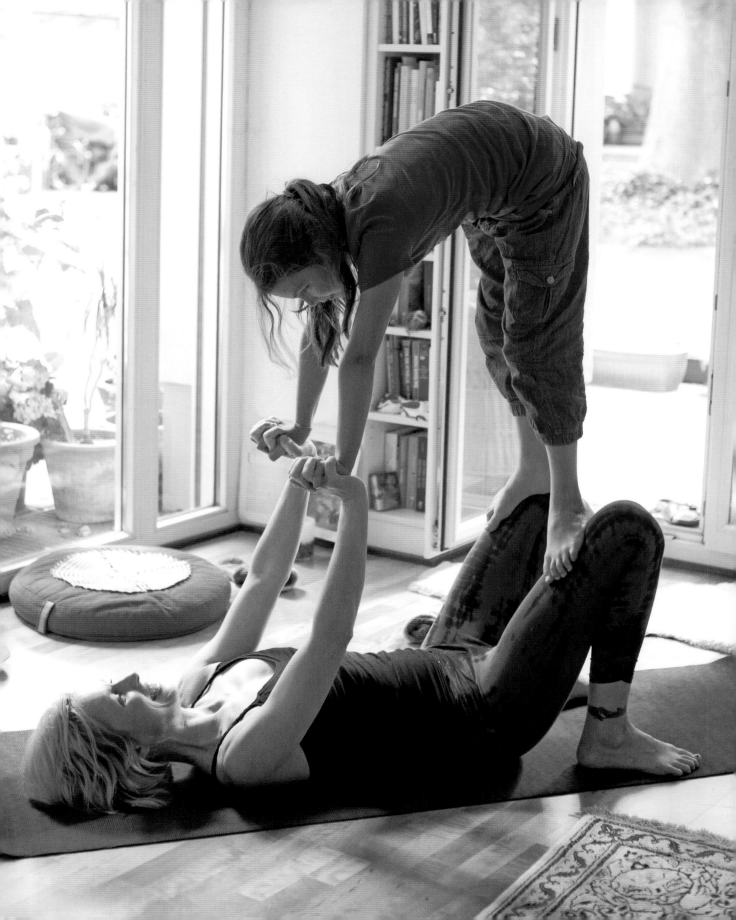

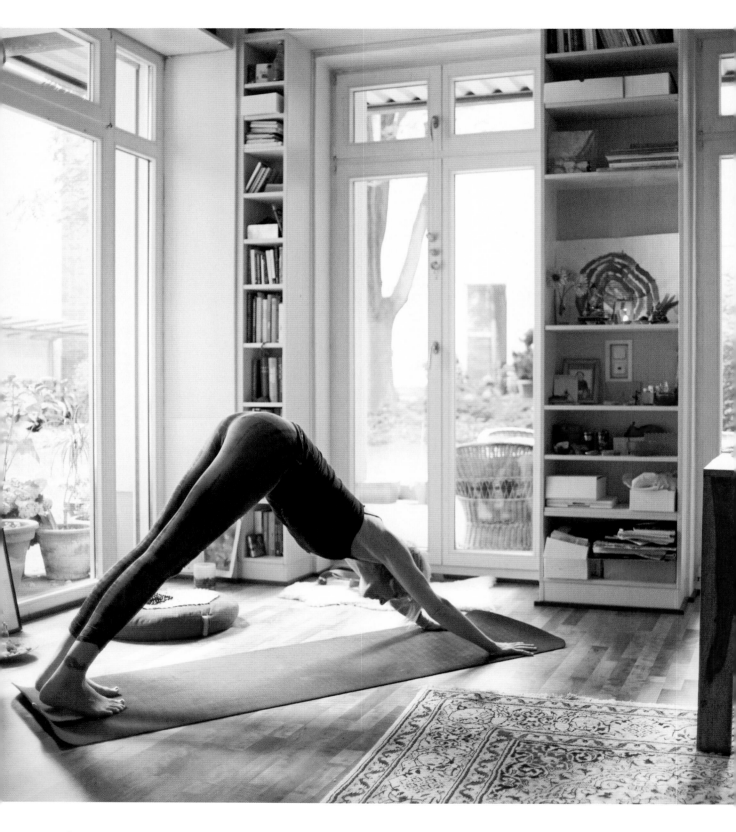

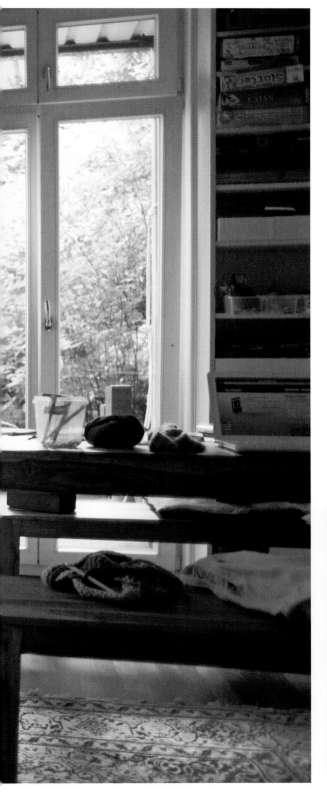

change every day: weather, food, amount of sleeping time, and many other things.

If I feel uninspired, there is the possibility to work on the asanas that need my full attention: Handstand, Full Pigeon, Hanumanasana, and Urdhva Dhanurasana. Going deeper in these poses teaches me a lot about how to align better—my body with my heart and mind, my bones, and my muscles.

I see my yoga mat as a laboratory: at home I can take my time to really understand the poses. In class, I like the Shakti energy, the one big breath together, the support of the others. But at home, I call my teachers and friends into my heart to support me in my willingness to understand what an asana wants from me and what it offers back to me. As a yoga teacher, it's important to develop more ideas of how to get into a pose. Instead of waiting for advice from an outer guru, my home practice connects me with my inner guru. It's yoga from the inside out. Sometimes I sit down in my practice and write my insights on the physical or emotional body. This helps me so much in understanding my students better.

As a modern woman with lots of jobs to do, I cannot imagine a life without yoga! It gives me strength and sensitivity in my behavior toward others and myself. It offers me equanimity and raises my radiance. And, I haven't been sick for the last ten years. It's good to trust in your own health!

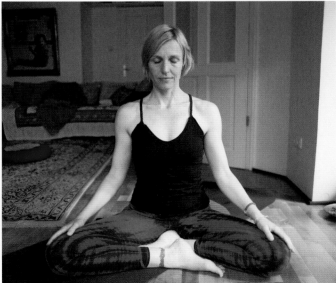

"Why do I practice? I am simply more creative, more humble, and more loving when I do."

Elena Brower

NEW YORK, NEW YORK | YOGA TEACHER/AUTHOR

Mama, teacher, speaker, and coauthor of *Art of Attention*, Elena has been influenced by several traditions, including Erich Schiffmann's Freedom Style Yoga, Rod Stryker's Para Yoga, and the Vedic meditation techniques of Thom Knoles.

At home, I have two spaces I practice in: my bedroom on my lamb's wool rug and my living room in the middle of whatever is going on. My bedroom is where I do my Kundalini *kriyas*, Halasana (Plow Pose), and sit for meditation. My living room is where I roll out my black mat and really practice asana. When the weather is nice, though, it's all about my roof. When I can get out there early enough, watching the sun rise over the East River from thirty-two floors up brings a lot of magic to my day.

Why do I practice? I am simply more creative, more humble, and more loving when I do. What helps

ELENA'S PRACTICE ADVICE

- I treat my entire house as a sacred space. Prior to practice, I clean up and take care of the space so it feels clear.

- Spend a few days or even weeks disposing of anything in your home that needs to be released (clothing, objects, etc.) with a patient eye toward creating a new sacred space for your yoga.

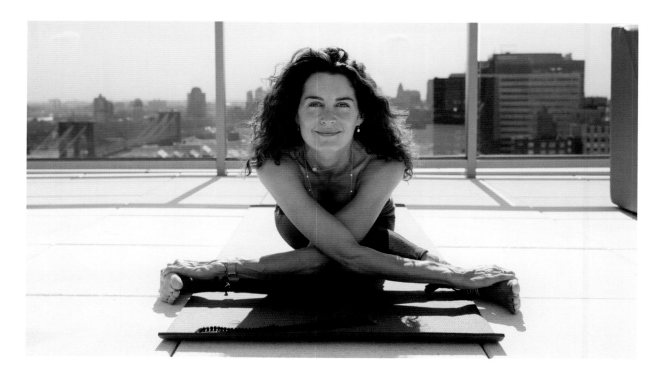

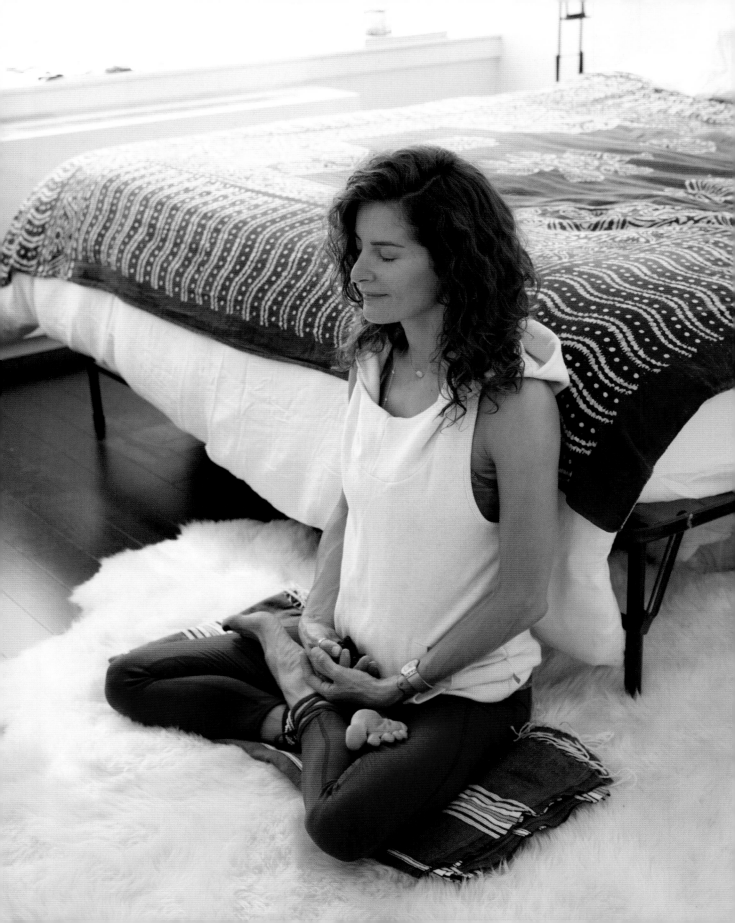

me get on my yoga mat even on those days I don't really want to? Sometimes my personal practice is as simple as Child's Pose. In really trying moments, that's enough to connect me to a prayerful state and begin a process of healing whatever needs to be recalibrated. My home practice always begins with a card reading: *Voyager Tarot*, Goddess cards, Angel cards, and now our new *Art of Attention* cards are my oracles. I'll choose one or two decks and pull from them, and use that inspiration for a word of the day, which I'll write on our miniature family chalkboard. Then I'll base my meditation, asana, and writing practice on that quality or reminder.

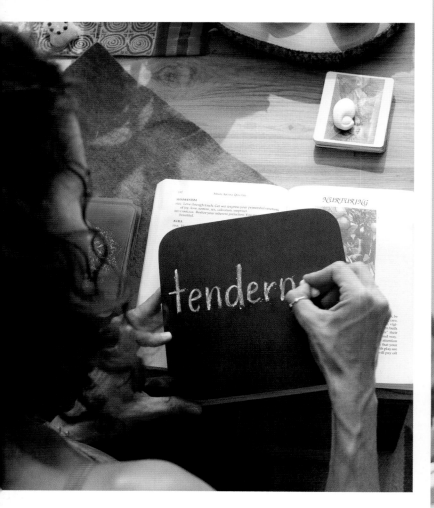

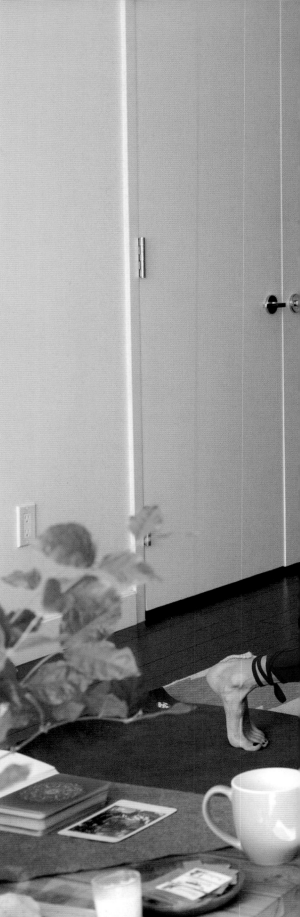

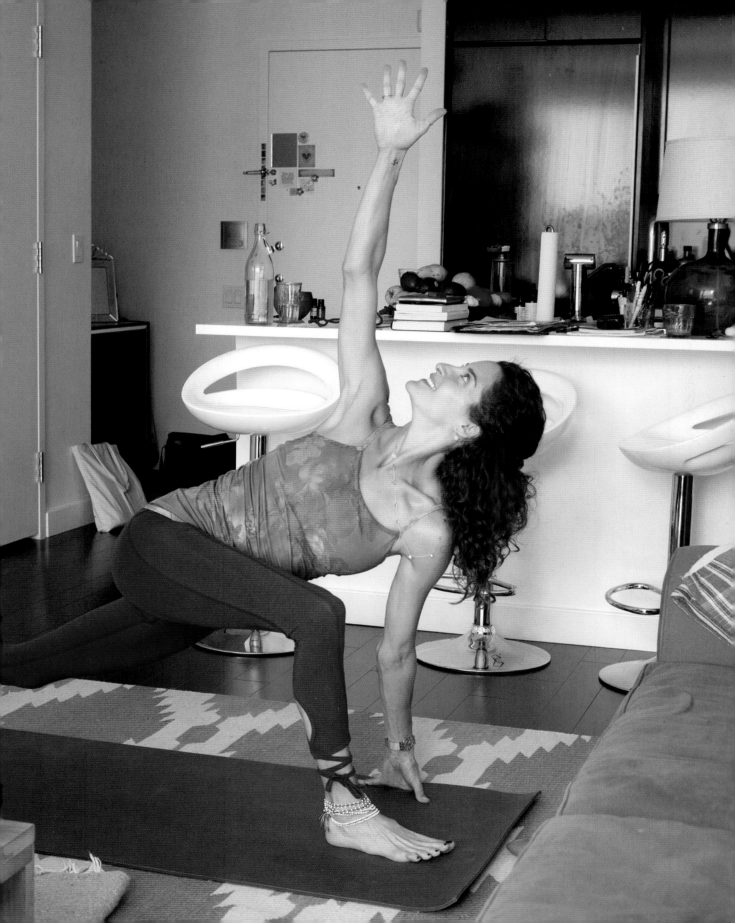

"I refer to my practice as life support. In every way, it supports and enhances my life."

Desiree Rumbaugh

ENCINITAS, CALIFORNIA | YOGA TEACHER

As a longtime student of Iyengar and Anusara yoga, Desiree blends playful humor with an authentic inquiry into the nature of being to help her Wisdom Warriors (yogis over fifty) discover their own power and beauty.

Since we are lucky to have a beautiful view of the ocean, I am mostly drawn to practice there, in front of the large window, looking out at the sea. I am inspired by nature and how the view changes according to the time of day and the seasons. There is enough space to share it with a few others as well, and sometimes this is how we engage with our guests if they are into yoga. If I need a quieter, cozier, more

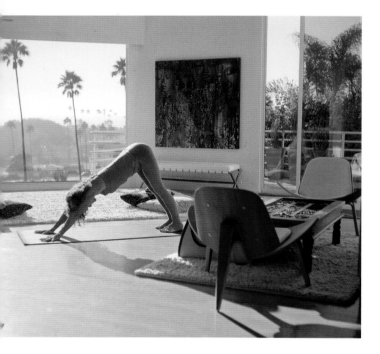

DESIREE'S PRACTICE ADVICE

🌼 Learn how to heal yourself with yoga at the same time you are learning to be stronger and more flexible. Once you learn how to heal your own ailments, you will be hooked on feeling great. To me, this is the best hook of all. It's more effective than sheer discipline or routine. Knowing that I have the power to heal my body and restore balance emotionally is what draws me to the practice every time.

private space, I will sometimes go downstairs to the guest bedroom and close the door.

My study and practice over the last three decades have shaped my view of life in every way. I have learned how to identify more with myself rather than only identifying with my human experience. This has given me more strength and power as I have had to deal with the unpredictable events of daily life here on Earth. This inner steadiness has been my life support, especially during the most traumatic experience of my life so far: my son's untimely passing, an unsolved murder, in 2003. I sometimes refer to my yoga practice as life support. In every way, it supports and enhances my life.

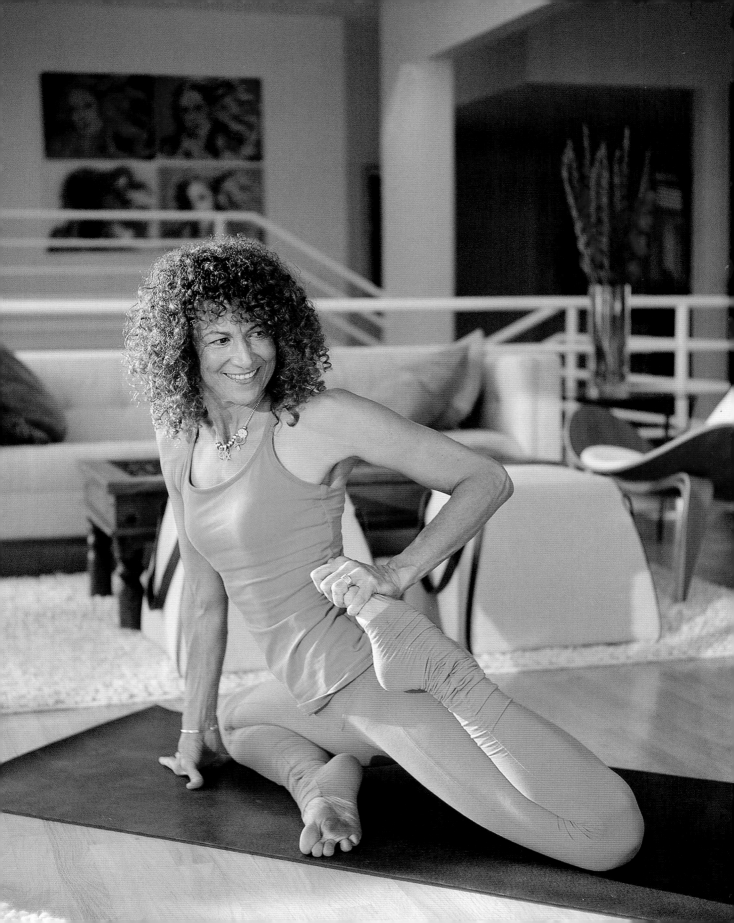

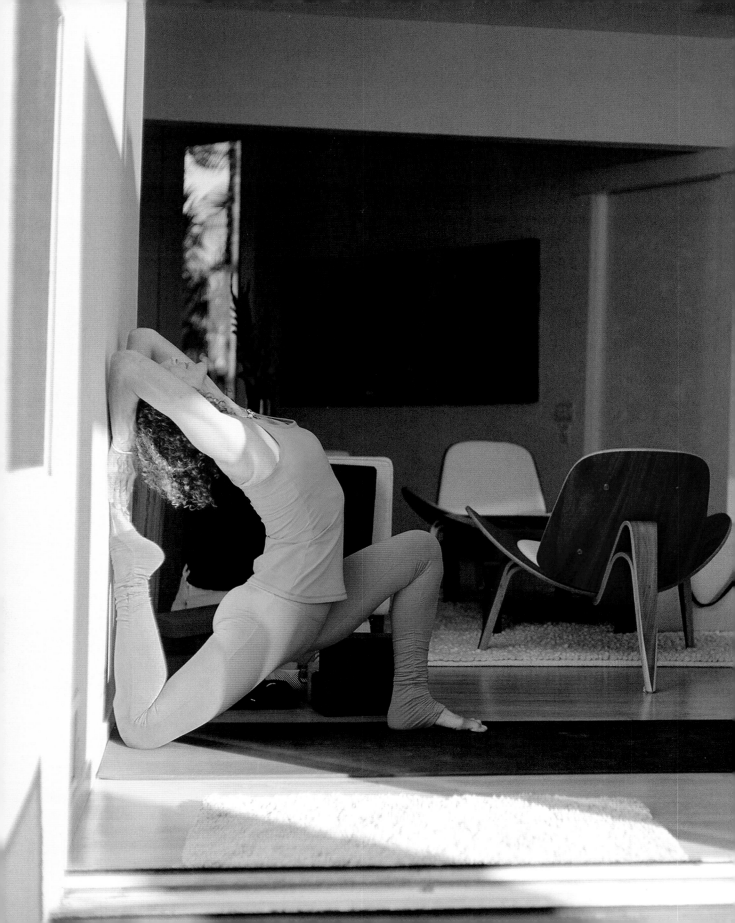

DESIREE'S SAMPLE PRACTICE

To get started, choose some music that inspires you. Then, go to your mat to either heal yourself or celebrate how great you feel at that moment. Begin with the idea of setting yourself free.

If your neck and shoulders are your tightest spots, do some stretches like these:

- Hold a belt above your head, separate your hands, and open your chest.

- Standing next to a wall, place one hand behind you against the wall and turn your body away in order to stretch tight pecs.

- Clasp your hands behind your back and bend over, allowing your shoulders to stretch and the blood to flow to your head.

Pay close attention to your breath during all of this and repeat the sequence a couple of times. The body needs and enjoys repetition.

For your lower back, focus on three areas: hamstrings (back of the thighs); quadriceps (front of the thighs); and gluteals (outer hips).

- Stretch your hamstrings by doing Uttanasana (Standing Forward Bends) with your legs hip-width apart or wider, bending your knees if you feel very stiff, and keeping your leg muscles engaged at all times.

- Stretch your outer hips and inner thighs with lunges, Eka Pada Galavasana (Figure Four Pose), and Malasana (Garland Pose).

- Do some standing stretches for your quadriceps. You can also do Bhekasana (Frog Pose): lie on your belly and bend one leg at a time, pulling it closer to your hip.

Repeat these stretches, watching your breath very closely. Hold each stretch and breathe, visualizing the muscle lengthening and becoming nourished.

After you have opened your shoulders and hips, take time to listen to your own guidance, moving from whatever knowledge you have of

poses you wish to try. Practice standing poses, seated poses, backbends, inversions, or arm balances according to what you have learned from your classes and workshops. Always close your practice with Savasana (Corpse Pose) or Viparita Karani (Legs-Up-the-Wall Pose). Be sure to take some time to sit and breathe in stillness to honor yourself.

Finally, bow to your inner teacher and your sacred space and move into your day with renewed awareness and a warm presence.

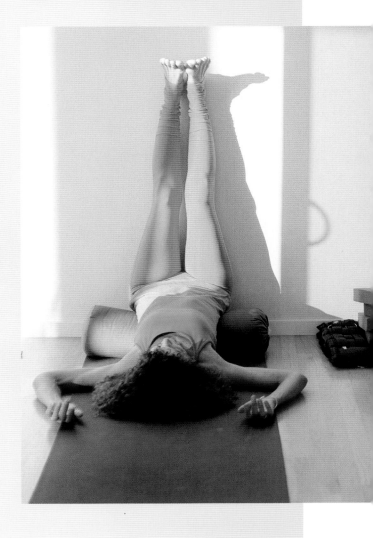

> *"My home practice is a very intimate time during the day to be just with myself."*

Detlev Alexander

BERLIN, GERMANY | YOGA TEACHER

Dancer, teacher, yogi, and Buddhist meditator, Detlev offers classes in Berlin and weeklong retreats throughout Europe. He is known to encourage everyone to become friends with themselves and to develop loving kindness and authenticity.

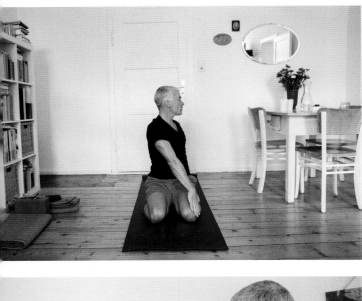

My home practice is a very intimate time during the day to be just with myself, seeing and meeting myself as I am in that given moment. It also allows me to practice the asanas I later want to teach, to embody those asanas and sequences until everything I want to teach is in every cell of my body. I feel a bit like a scientist, observing every little movement in my body and mind. That way I become familiar with myself, with my personal habits. I experience moments of freshness and wakefulness, which then show up in my everyday life and also while I'm teaching yoga.

DETLEV'S PRACTICE ADVICE

- As soon as you start to do yoga at home, your practice will definitely change. It will become *your* practice and not the practice of your teacher or somebody else. This is one of the most important steps toward freedom—and isn't freedom the ultimate goal of yoga?

- If you're just beginning a home practice, start small. Rather than a full 90-minute yoga practice, do just 5 or 10 minutes. Begin with some poses you like to practice and stick with them for a while.

- Commit to a certain time and place, and create a space you like to come back to every day.

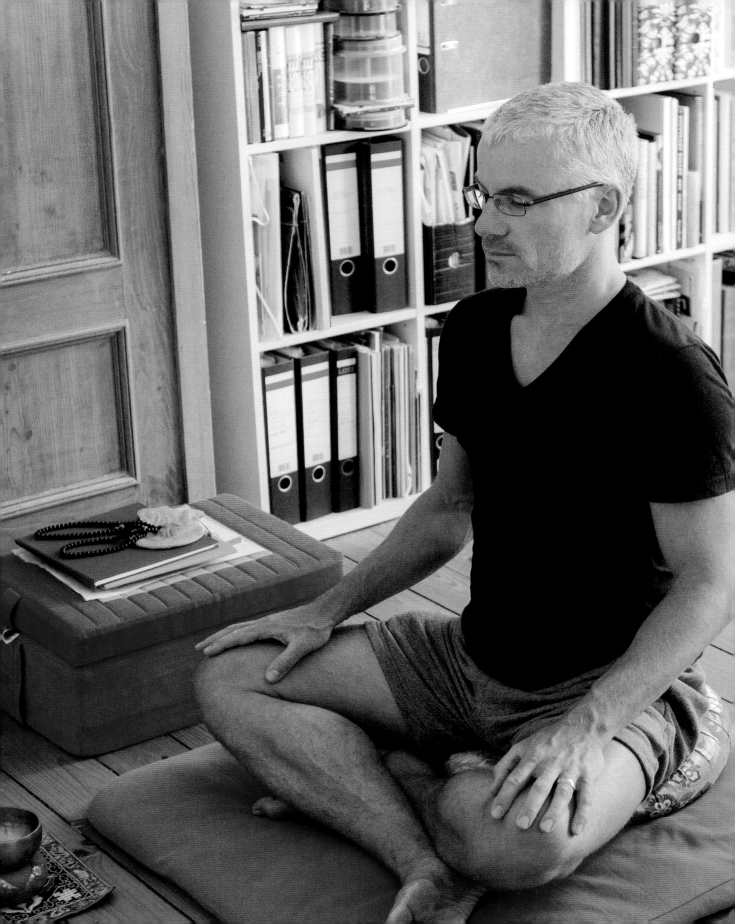

> *"Our home is our sacred nurturing space where we embrace everything we do as our practice."*

Jai Uttal & Nubia Teixeira

FAIRFAX, CALIFORNIA | MUSICIAN • YOGA TEACHER/DANCER

Joyfulness, kindness, and deep wisdom come together when performing artist, musician, and storyteller Jai interweaves his devotional kirtan with the asanas, mantras, mudras, and pranayamas of Nubia's multicultural Bhakti Nova Yoga.

Our intention is to bring sacredness into every moment of our lives. We have pictures and statutes of gods and goddesses on every wall and surface of our home, but we know that sacredness is really created by love. So we try to be super kind, caring, and affectionate to each other all the time. Often, the three of us just melt into a big puddle of love—on the bed, the couch, or even the yoga mat. We do

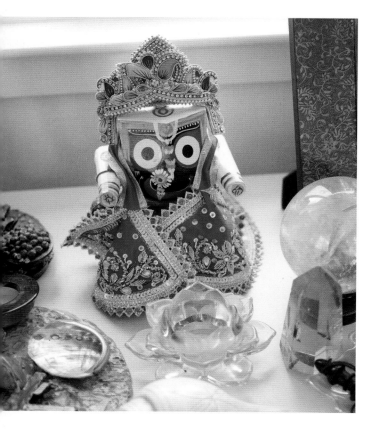

JAI'S PRACTICE ADVICE

- Start with baby steps, and be consistent.
- Be kind to yourself and don't judge yourself. We have everything we need within us to nurture our personal and intimate relationship to God. Our moods are the multicolored expressions of our hearts, which are mirrors of the divine heart. So please, don't refrain . . . let your voice and spirit expand in all directions.

yoga in every room—*japa* (mantra) in our son Ezra's room; asana, music, and dance in the living room; *Hanuman Chalisa* (hymn to Hanuman) in the prayer room; kirtan cooking and dishwashing in the kitchen; and divine sleeping in the bedroom. Our home is our sacred nurturing space where we embrace everything we do as our practice.

JAI: My home practice consists of prayers, mantras, and music, with an occasional asana thrown in for flavor. Our house is quite small so we've done our best to turn every nook and cranny into an altar. Everywhere we look in our home we are reminded of God. Although I have a beautiful altar and prayer room in a small downstairs cave-like room where I pray and do *puja* (offerings to the deity) every evening, my favorite place to practice is on the living room couch, where I sit with my guitar and sing songs of love and longing.

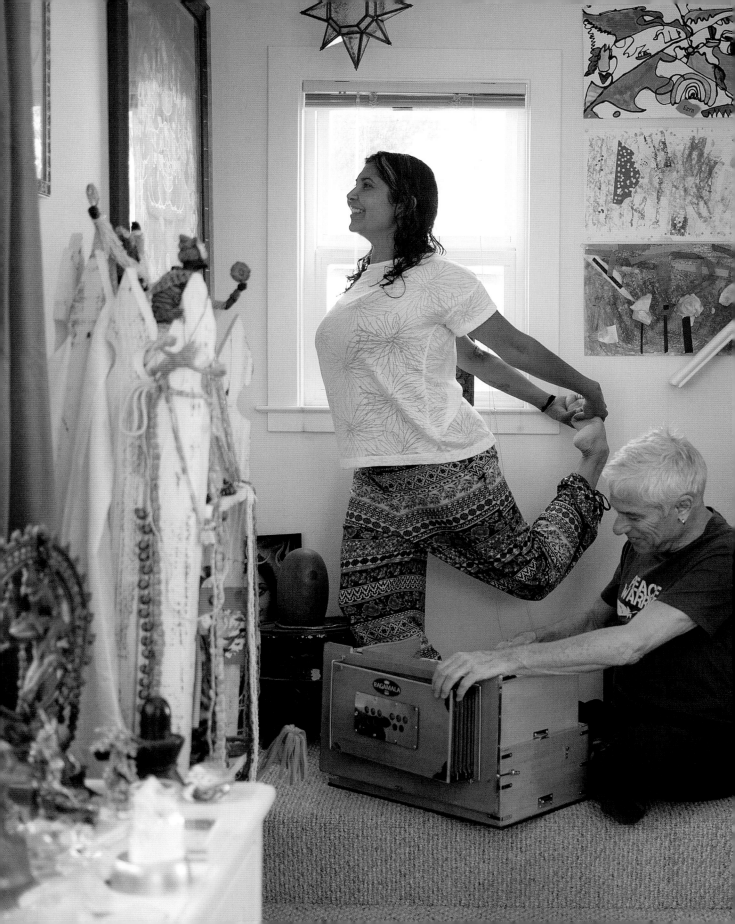

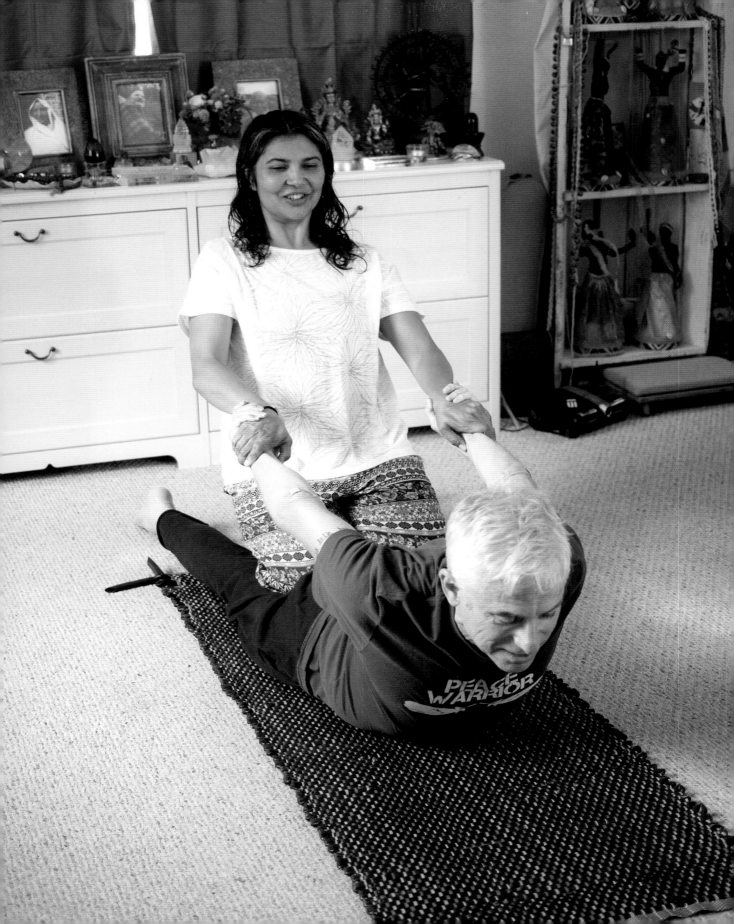

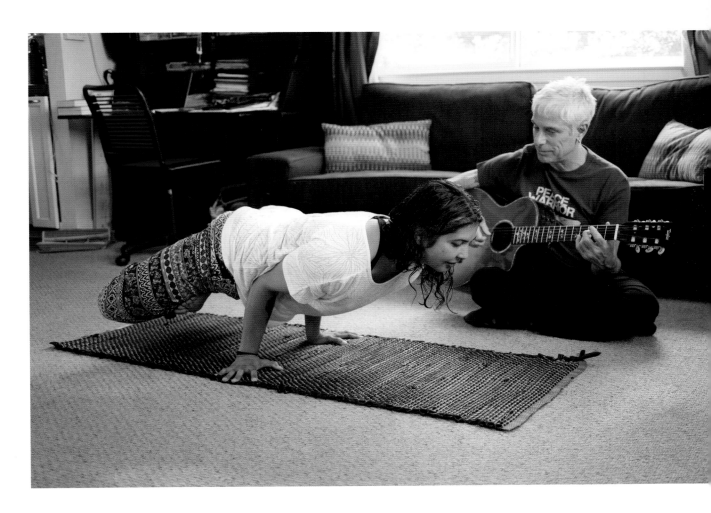

NUBIA: My home practice starts when I open my eyes and roll out of bed into Child's Pose, crawl my way up to standing, and walk up the stairs to our kitchen and living-room space. I warm up and drink a big glass of ginger water, and then start my *kriya* practices—*neti*, *nauli*, and *trataka*. Then I brush my teeth, wash my face, and go light a candle on our living-room altar to say good morning to our gurus and ask for guidance for the day. I make a point to wake up early and have the house just for me. After prayers and my chai, I move into my asana and pranayama practice.

JAI: My life's journey has seen many mountains and valleys. When I met my guru, Neem Karoli Baba, at nineteen years of age, he tied a cord to my heart, connecting us for eternity. But this did not stop me from taking many wrong turns until I found myself lost and

NUBIA'S PRACTICE ADVICE

- ❀ Make it as simple and as playful as you can, so it is something you want to get back to every day. Have a practice plan, but leave some room for spontaneity.

- ❀ Follow your inner guide and adhere to your inner alignment, rather than what is imposed by others.

alone in what seemed to be a dark and empty world. Nonetheless, the practice of kirtan and the repetition of God's names, as he instructed, maintained that lifesaving cord. So many times when I thought I was drowning, remembrance of my guru and the sacred names pulled me back to the shore. Really, I feel that this was all due to his grace, both the darkness and the light. Remembering and surrendering over and over again to that grace is truly the heart of my practice.

NUBIA: Yoga in my life equals grace. I grew up in Brazil in a very poor family, and there seemed to be little potential for prosperity and expansion. At the age of sixteen, I found yoga to be the savior that I was waiting for. I still wonder, did I find yoga, or did yoga find me? I started teaching when I was eighteen and so many doors opened, internally and externally. A vast richness of possibilities and qualities unfolded within me through the wealth of the ancient teachings and connections. I feel like my life has been blessed with light, grace, and love.

JAI: Some days I dive deeply into my practices and practicing, other days the time spent is minimal, but I have a bottom line: a day doesn't go by when I don't do my evening prayers and *puja*. I was told by my Indian mother to "practice and wait for grace," so I am trying to do my part with faith and patience and sure knowledge that grace will come.

NUBIA: Not doing my practice equals feeling pain and causing pain. Yoga and dance balance my entire being and without that balance I stumble and temporarily lose my connection with Spirit. I cherish this connection so much, not just for myself, but also for what it allows me to give to my family and students. The desire to serve is what inspires me to keep practicing.

JAI & NUBIA: It is by practicing solo that we find a sense of our own unique expression, and the special gifts that are ours to share. Then, when we reenter our community, with full and overflowing hearts, our energy is contagious and lights up everyone around us.

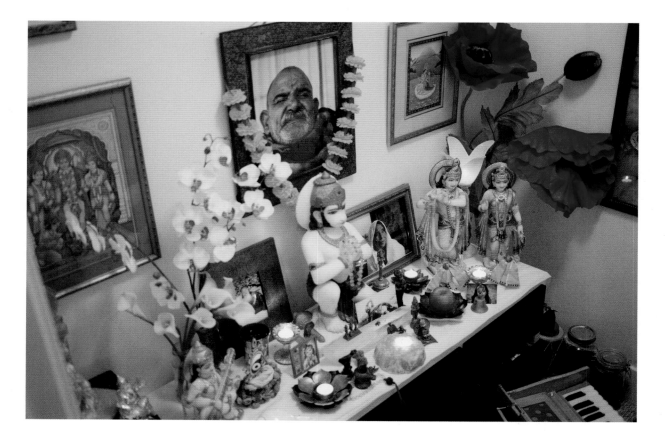

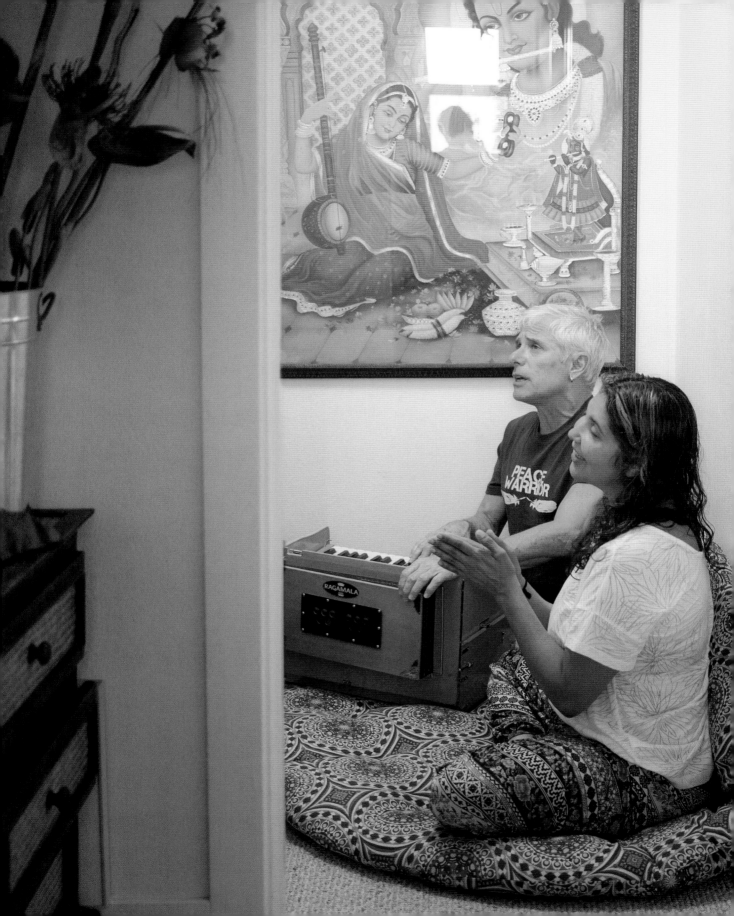

> *"My approach to creating a home practice is rooted in the methodology of process design."*

Erica Jago

MAUI, HAWAII | YOGA TEACHER/DESIGNER

An accomplished designer, author, and yoga teacher, Erica leads classes and retreats using vinyasa and Kundalini yoga to help students master a profound love in their attitudes, emotional experiences, and in their relationship to their bodies.

Using the touchpoints of sound and smell inspire my spiritual practice. Turning on some music will point me to playfulness, and lighting incense, especially frankincense and myrrh, will bring me back into my softness. I view these effortless gestures as a way of putting a signal out to something much larger than myself, that I'm willing to engage, that my body is their container, and then I eagerly await the assistance.

My approach to creating a home practice is very much rooted in the methodology of process design. I begin by drawing a sequence out graphically using what I call Asanaglyphs, symbolic line art that allows me to form a narrative and see the poetic nature of the practice. I record the flow from pose to pose, getting all the physical, mental, and emotional aspects of my alignment to move together simultaneously and with a particular theme—for example, opening the heart. Therefore, the home practice is thoughtfully designed to get familiar with this alignment and what it is like to hold the heart in this space for a few breaths at a time. The best part of this process is that I'm documenting the ideas and inspirations visually, which for me is a very powerful communication tool for self-study and a great way to look back and reflect on my growth.

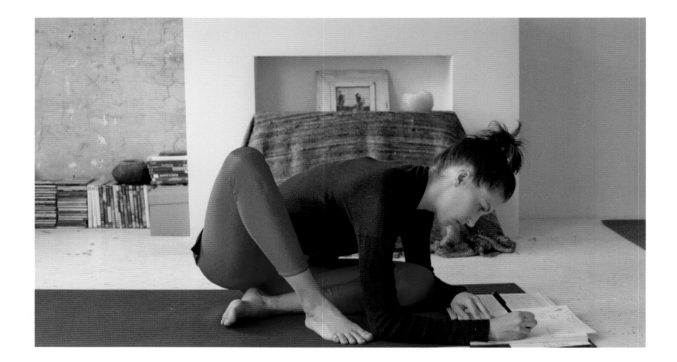

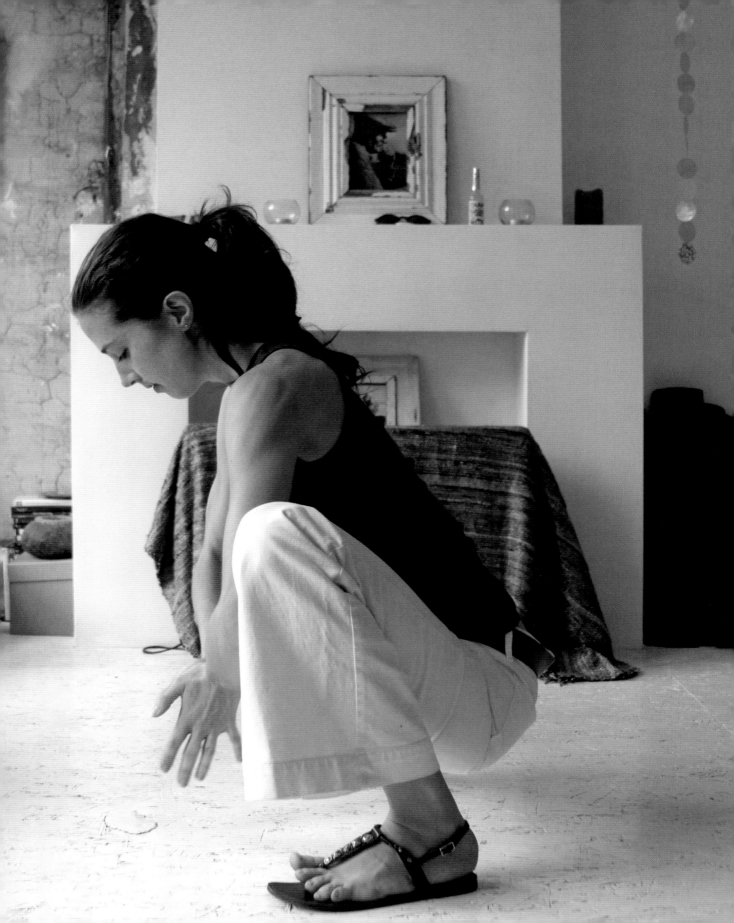

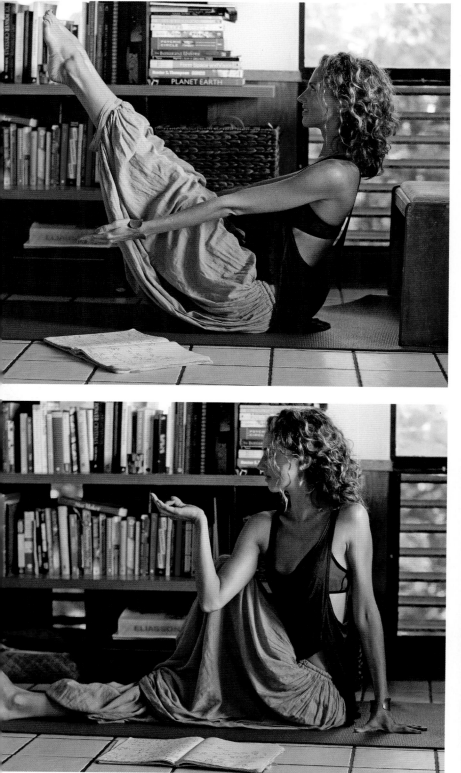

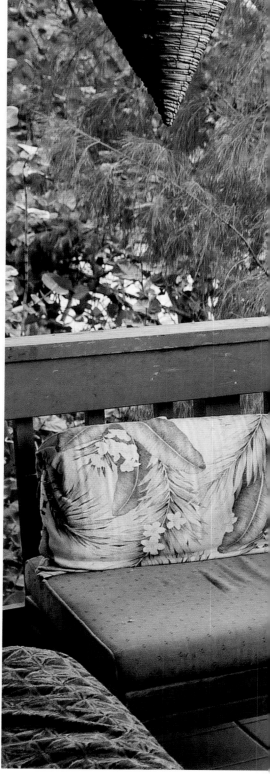

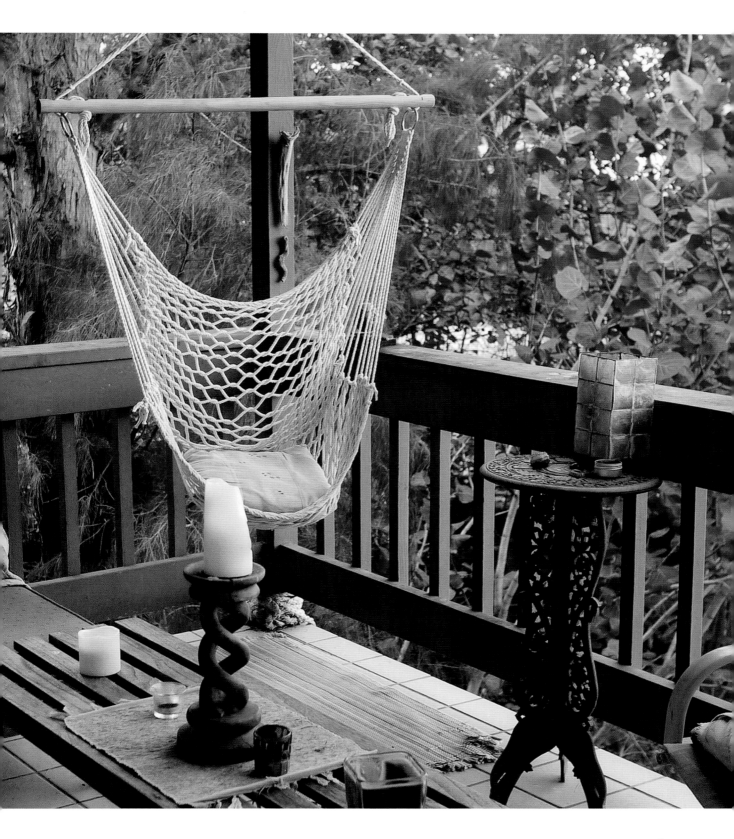

"The inner teachings of yoga bring creativity, passion, and the sacred into the everyday."

Shiva Rea

MALIBU, CALIFORNIA | YOGA TEACHER/AUTHOR

Creator of Prana Flow yoga and author of *Tending the Heart Fire: Living in Flow with the Pulse of Life,* Shiva is known for bringing the roots of yoga alive for modern practitioners in creative, dynamic, and transforming ways.

I started making altars on the beach near where we lived when I was just a little girl. Later, when I was fourteen, I gravitated toward yoga as a way to make sense of the yogic name my father had given me. At first, I would seek out the most light-filled corner of our old Victorian house in Memphis, Tennessee, and practice there. But after a while, the Mississippi River—which was just a few blocks away—called to me and became my favorite spot to meditate and pray during my turbulent teenaged years.

These days, my entire house is filled with altars and a sense of blessed intimacy permeates every room.

The little altars in my kitchen, on my writing desk, on the dining table, out on the deck, in my bedroom, in the closet, and even in the bathtub dissolve the boundaries between the yoga of practice and the yoga of life. As a result, I am better able to fulfill my mission as a yoga teacher/householder, which is to bring an element of "living vinyasa" to the cycles and flow of each day. The inner teachings of yoga, as depicted by my altars, bring creativity, passion, and a sense of the sacred into the everyday and reflect the gratefulness and connection I feel to my own body. My body becomes my altar, and my home, the body's temple.

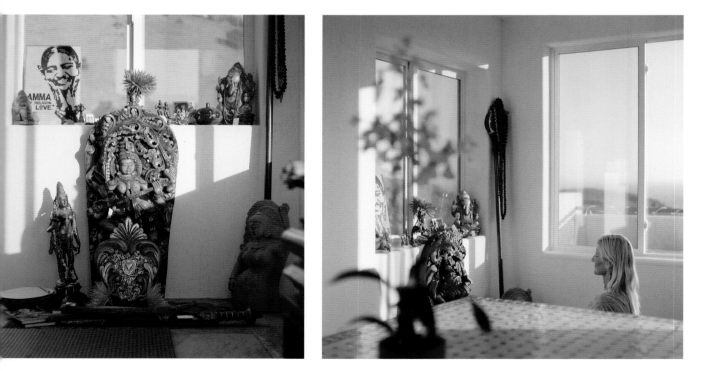

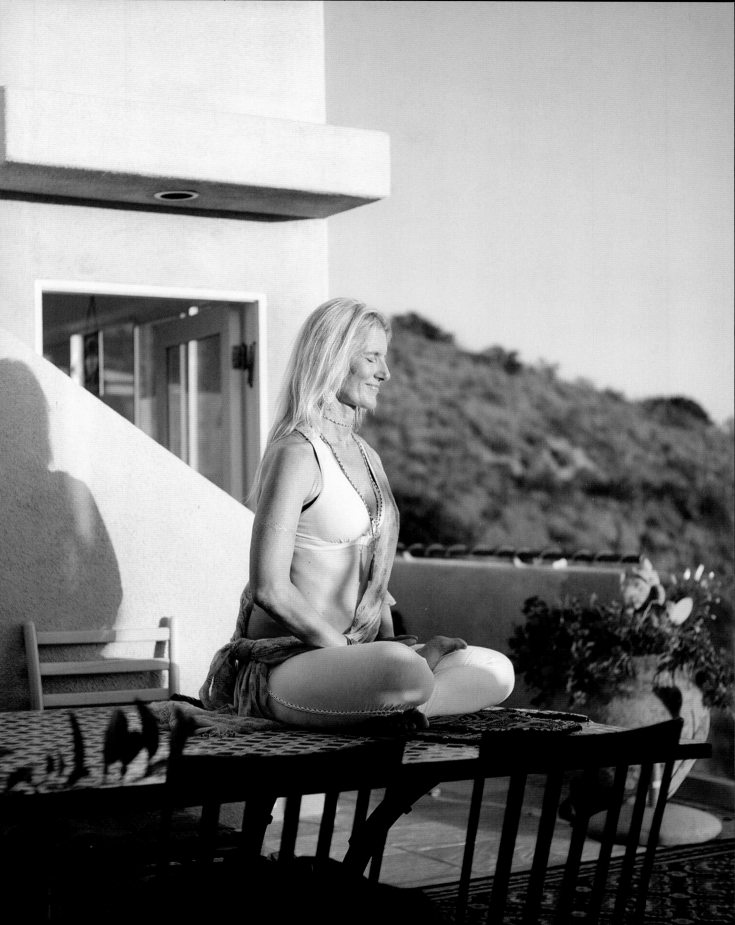

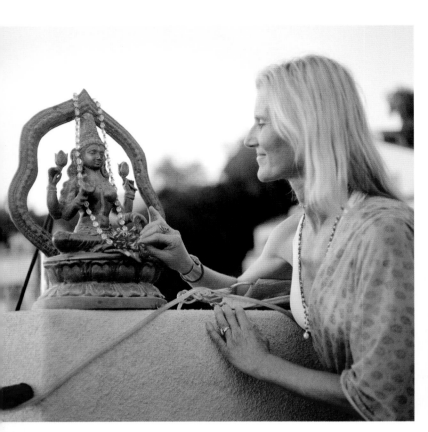

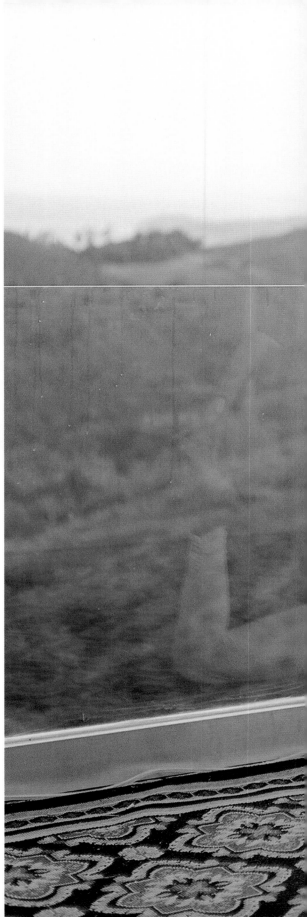

The ability to attune myself with sunrise and sunset is one of the main practices in yoga that I have brought to my home practice. For the first time in my life, I can see the sunrise from a window. So now my morning practice space is in the kitchen and dining-room area, where I can see the sun come up behind the Santa Monica Mountains. I awaken for sunrise meditation or early morning mantra and then I write before the world comes alive.

At sunset, I usually meander to the outside deck, where Solstice Canyon becomes the altar as I watch the color of the sky transform. I find I prefer to move in the afternoon, and sunset has this way of melting the day within one's body and mind. I find my spine goes deeper in backbends at sunset. I used to love teaching classes at that time, but now all business stops so I can savor life in any way possible—yoga, meditation, creative arts, reflection, cooking, lying around, going outside to enjoy the prana of the earth altar. I end up working odd hours to make sure I'm not missing the times of the day that my home practice thrives.

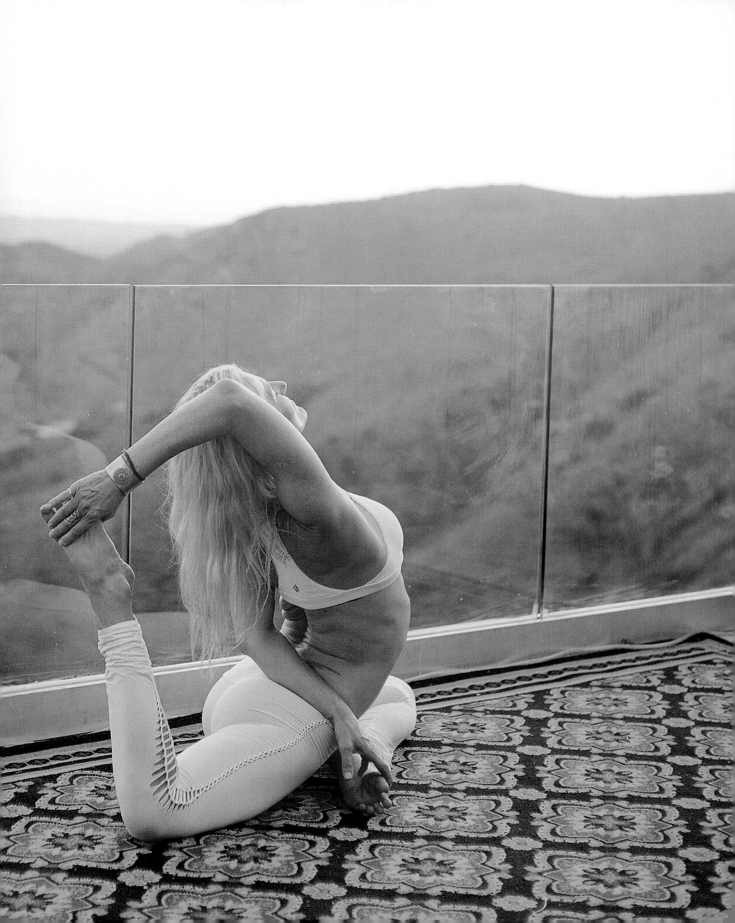

"Faith gives me the motivation and curiosity to explore myself through practice."

Jules Febre

NEW YORK, NEW YORK | YOGA TEACHER

Born and raised on New York City's Lower East Side, Jules began studying yoga in India when he was only thirteen. These days, this Jivamukti teacher offers yoga classes worldwide and heads up operations for Jivamukti, Inc., in New York.

My teachers and students are the biggest instigators of my practice. I have felt something powerful transferred to me from my teachers in the form of guided instructions that bring clarity. I have faith in the words of my teachers that I am more than an individual simply trying to get by in the world.

That faith gives me the motivation and the curiosity to explore myself through practice. Knowing that I have chosen to get up in front of people and teach means yoga can't be about just theory. Wanting to share from a place of experiential knowledge pushes me to keep going.

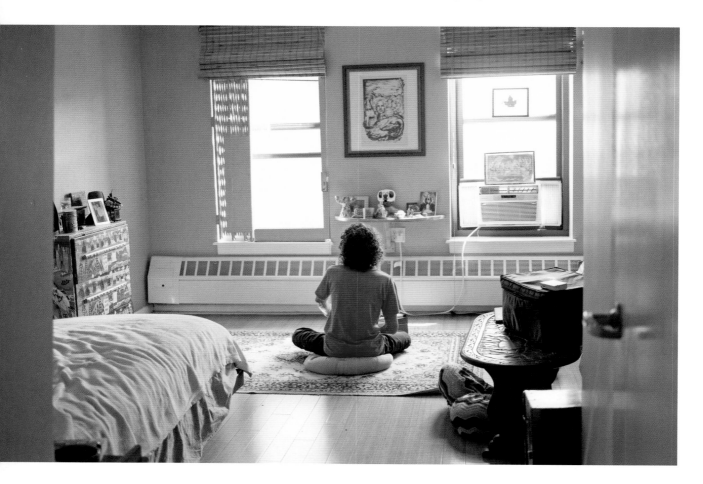

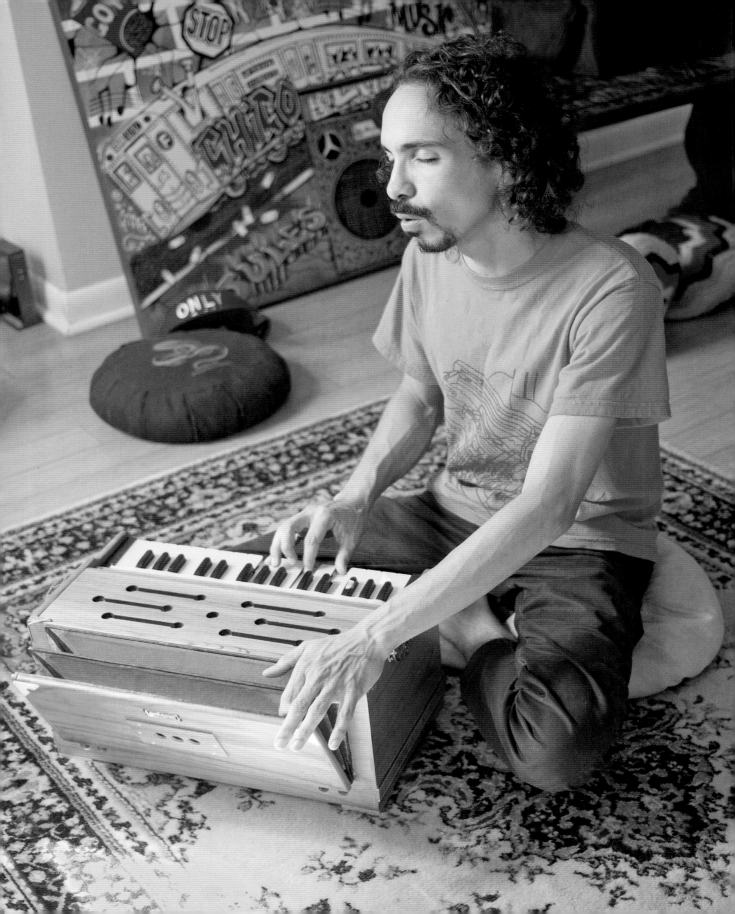

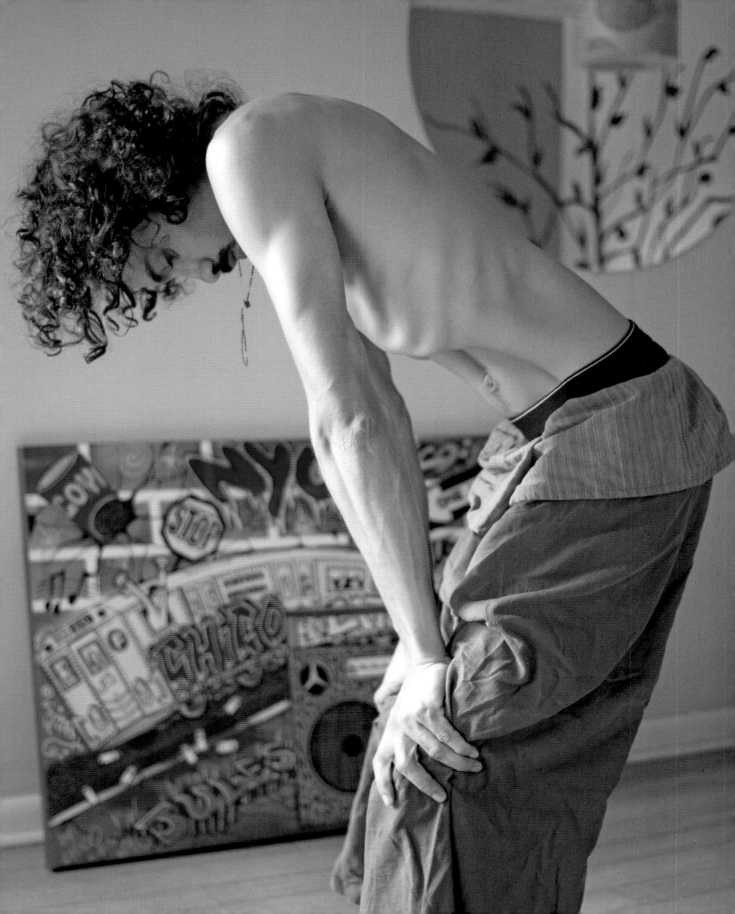

I can't really dedicate a separate room for my yoga practice, since I do not have one. Instead, I try to make the whole of the apartment suitable for practice. It's a bit like my apartment changes clothes—for city dwelling sometimes and then for yoga practice. I move most everything out of the way and out come the yoga props.

The practice itself changes based on what my mind and body need and that can be quite a challenge for me, because I don't usually want to do the things I most need. My practice often begins with an internal dialogue where I sit quietly and allow what is needed to rise up. Then I have to summon the courage to actually manifest it. Sometimes it takes longer than I would like to admit.

Lately, my practice has included a lot of singing as I play the harmonium—often chants to different aspects of the Divine both in English and Sanskrit. My practice can also include reading; sometimes from the ancient texts, like the *Bhagavad Gita*, *Yoga Sutra*, the Koran, or the Bible, other times from the writing of great contemporary teachers. No matter what or how I decide to practice, I make it a point to start my day in a special way, set an intention to do my best to be happy and grateful for what I have, and remember that my happiness is intricately entwined with the happiness of those around me.

I've also found that cooking for me is very meditative and gives me a chance to create something that nourishes the body and something I can use as an offering. In many of the bhakti traditions, food is offered up to a deity. For me, that is a little too abstract. I like to invite friends over as often as possible, create a *satsang* (a gathering of people interested in yogic pursuits), and feed them. Cooking for myself is a nice practice, too, but I find it easier and often more rewarding when cooking for others. In fact, if I don't feel like doing a practice first thing in the morning, I will often make a large, delicious meal while chanting.

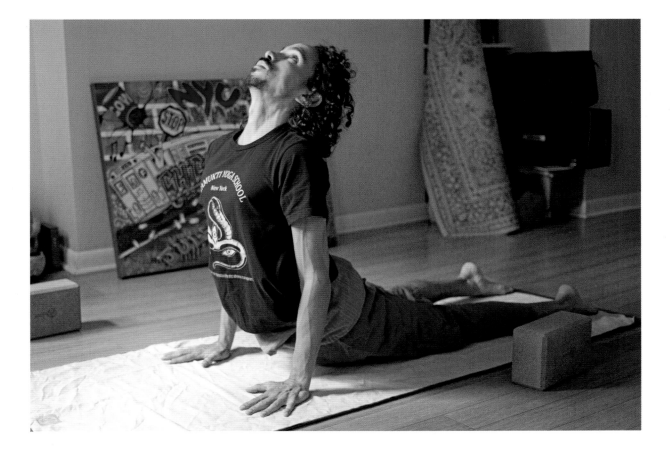

> *"My practice is all about being online, being wirelessly connected to the infinity of mind."*

Erich Schiffmann

LOS ANGELES, CALIFORNIA | YOGA TEACHER

For Erich, creator of Freedom Style Yoga, yoga is a way of moving into stillness in order to experience the truth of who you are; it is an invitation to listen inwardly for guidance and then dare to do as you are prompted to do.

I had a disciplined structure for my practice, which was great for about six or seven years. Loved, loved, loved it. But then I loved it less and less. No one was saying what the next step was. All I knew was I was enjoying my practice less. The whole structured discipline wasn't holding me like it did initially. For a couple of years, I was confused because I thought all those years of disciplined practice were going down the tubes. I didn't love it *and* I hated that I didn't love it!

If only someone had told me that if the disciplined structure really works, it will dissolve. If someone had said that, it would have saved me so much anxiety. The new discipline became listening for inner guidance,

and then, at that point, I suddenly didn't need the outward structure. I had inner discipline.

Years ago—in the 1970s in Pune, India—B. K. S. Iyengar was telling everyone to be very disciplined, but when I went early in the morning to watch him practice, Iyengar wasn't doing "disciplined." He was being guided from within. Now my practice is all about being online, being wirelessly connected to the infinity of mind, and daring to do that. So, when I go into my yoga room, it's more like . . . totally fun! I do exactly what I feel like doing.

We have a little add-on to the garage, away from the house and the street, with props, mats, and a sound

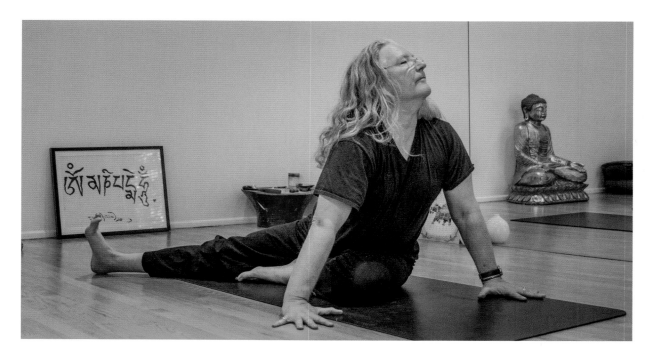

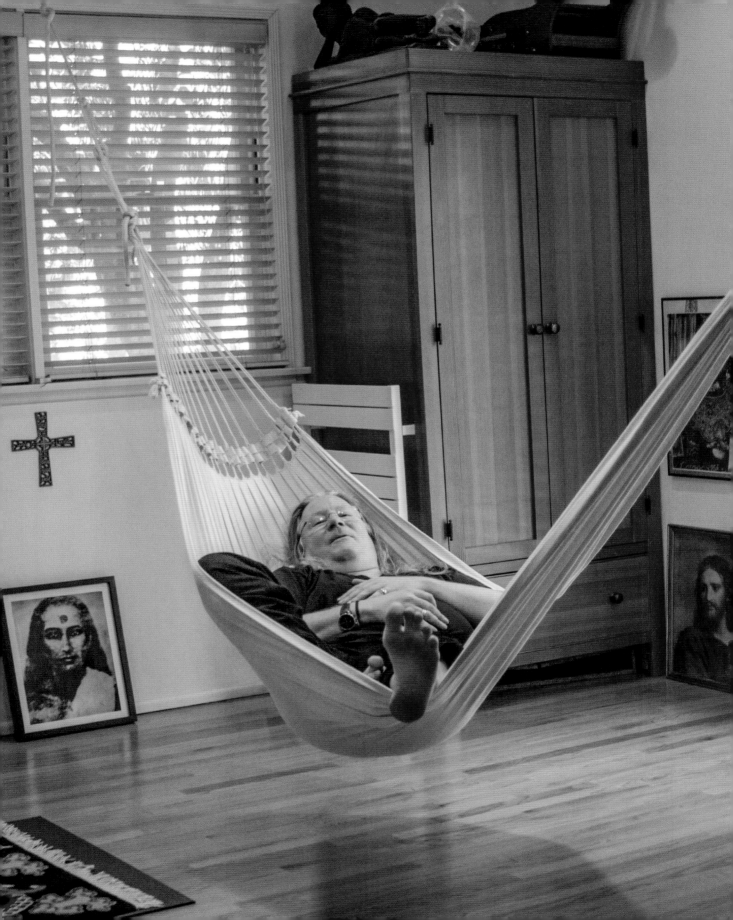

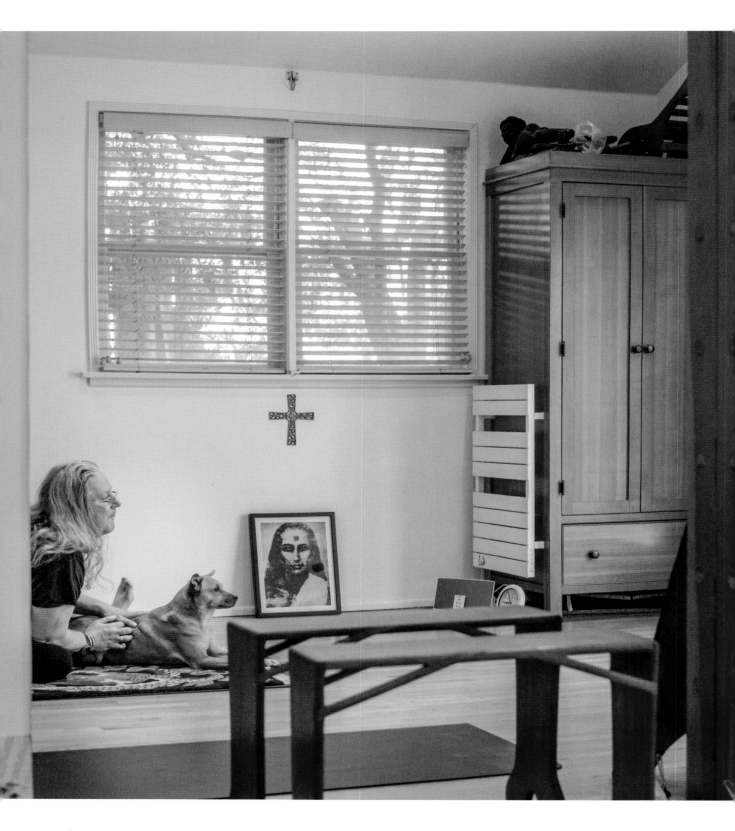

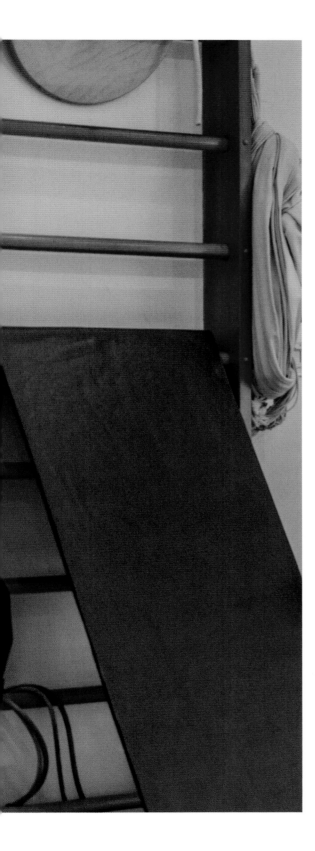

system. I go in there and I meditate first, but I've already meditated a bunch by that point! Then I do asana from 5:00 to 7:00 p.m. I have a notebook and a pen with me, and a tape recorder. If it feels like something special is happening, I turn the video camera on. And then I listen to what I should do. I'm in class with the Infinite. I'm down here taking notes. One thing leads to the next, and creates some interesting transitions.

I practice as long as it feels right. If don't feel like practicing, I don't. It's all about listening for inner guidance. If it doesn't come, then I don't do it. Most of the time, though, I go in. The practice is being wirelessly connected to the Infinite, daring you to do what feels right to you. It makes sense to trust yourself at a certain point.

ERICH'S PRACTICE ADVICE

- Find yourself a space to practice in. The place that is waiting for you should be nice, especially if you have difficulty practicing. If it's not to your liking, you'll have more reasons not to practice.

- Find poses you like to do, because then you might also do the ones you don't like.

- Rather than coming to the mat sporadically, use your enthusiasm to practice consistently, but be gentle—don't use force or control.

- One way of getting yourself to do your home practice is to invite your friends over. Everyone can do their own thing!

- If you're a beginner, do what your teacher taught you, but as you do it, start to get into it a little bit more, with a few change-it-up moments. You'll begin to deviate from the prescribed pattern. The energy will start moving you differently and then you have to be brave enough to let the energy guide you, making new shapes. Deviate from the pattern, and then pretty soon your practice will become this big-old deviation until it's no longer a deviation—it's you!

"Only by regular practice do we begin to find the road back home to ourselves."

Krishna Das

NYACK, NEW YORK | MUSICIAN

Krishna, affectionately known as KD, blends the musical and spiritual traditions of the East with the voice of the West to create kirtan, devotional call-and-response chanting that leads us home to our true state of being.

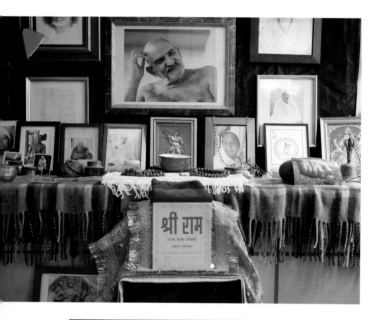

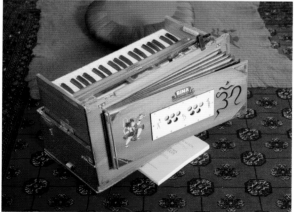

When I practice, I sit at my altar. All my teachers are there (in picture form as well as Essence Presence). This is where I sing when I am home and where I practice letting go and remembering. All the photos on my altar are of great beings I have met, a couple of them only in dreams, as they left the body long ago. Just hanging out with them deepens my practice because they are always here and present. We are the ones who aren't here! We invite the presence of God or the great saints to enter into our heart and take a seat at our altar. It is they who create the sacredness of the space.

My practice is the only thing that has saved me. As Saint Paul wrote, "By grace was I saved through faith."

KD'S PRACTICE ADVICE

- It is by repetition that we train ourselves. Through repetition, we get familiar with how it feels to be less obsessive and crazed and stressed. So only by regular practice do we begin to find the road back home to ourselves. If our physical home becomes a helper in that, it is a wonderful thing.

- I try to be real in whatever I do and not fool myself—at least for 1 minute every day!

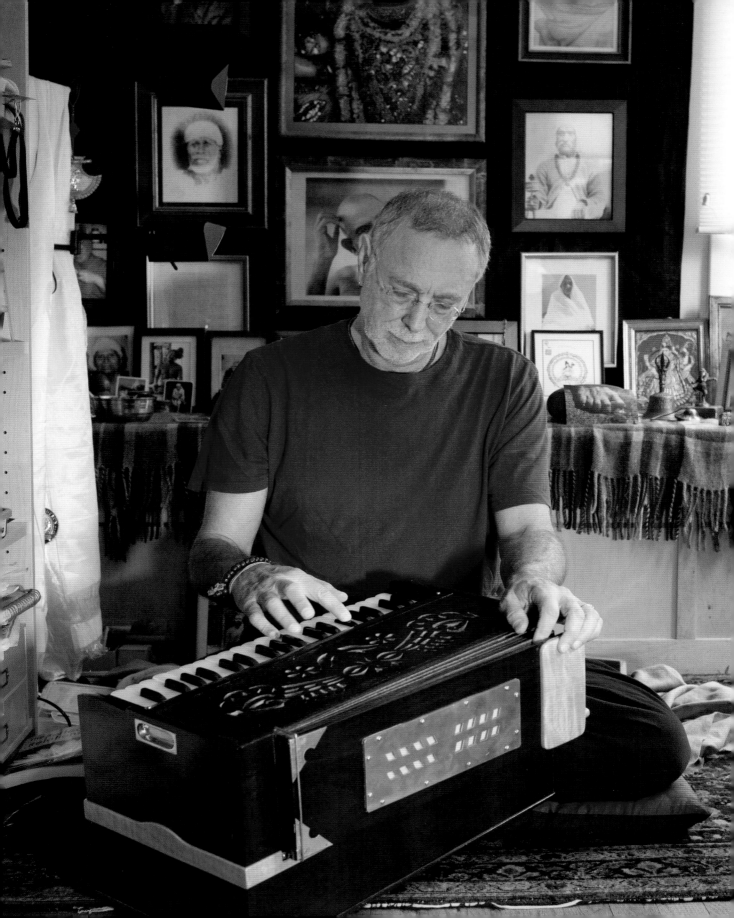

Margi Young

SAN FRANCISCO, CALIFORNIA | YOGA TEACHER

Margi, a San Francisco OM yoga teacher who teaches classes and workshops worldwide, sheepishly admits that there's a mental and physical journey she has to take between thinking "it's time to practice" and rolling out her mat.

There is absolutely nothing that I love more than to be on my mat exploring my body and breath. But, in the spirit of *satya* (truthfulness), I must admit that most days it's a struggle to practice at home. Why? First, I'm not a morning person. I know the ancient yogis say that we have the ability to change ourselves and create new *samskaras* (patterns), but every time I force myself to get up early, I fall back to sleep on my mat. I finally decided that it's OK not to practice in the morning and that's a samskara I can accept.

Second, practicing in my house is challenging for me. When I teach retreats and trainings away from my "normal life" of computers, family, work, dishes, and shopping—when the only things on the agenda are yoga, teaching, and eating—my personal practice is an uncomplicated delight. But when I'm at home, there's a mental and physical journey I have to take between the thought, "It's time to practice," and rolling out my mat. Once I finally get to that point, here are some things that help me practice.

I practice anytime from 8:00 a.m. to 11:00 p.m., but I can usually sink into a deep practice with a lot of restorative poses. I set a timer and commit to a set amount of time, and it doesn't matter whether it's 15 minutes or 90 minutes. That timer sets a very clear boundary and helps me to commit to the time on my mat. I keep a notebook next to my mat. When I think of tasks during my practice, instead of popping off my

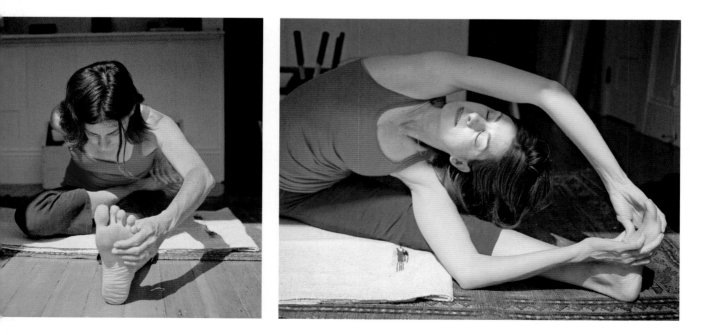

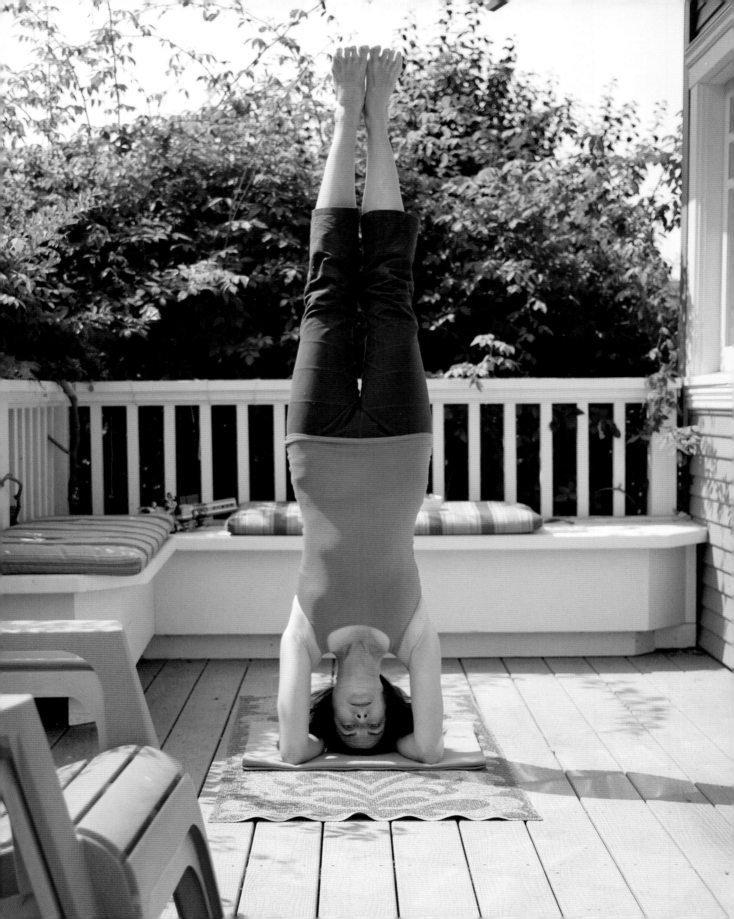

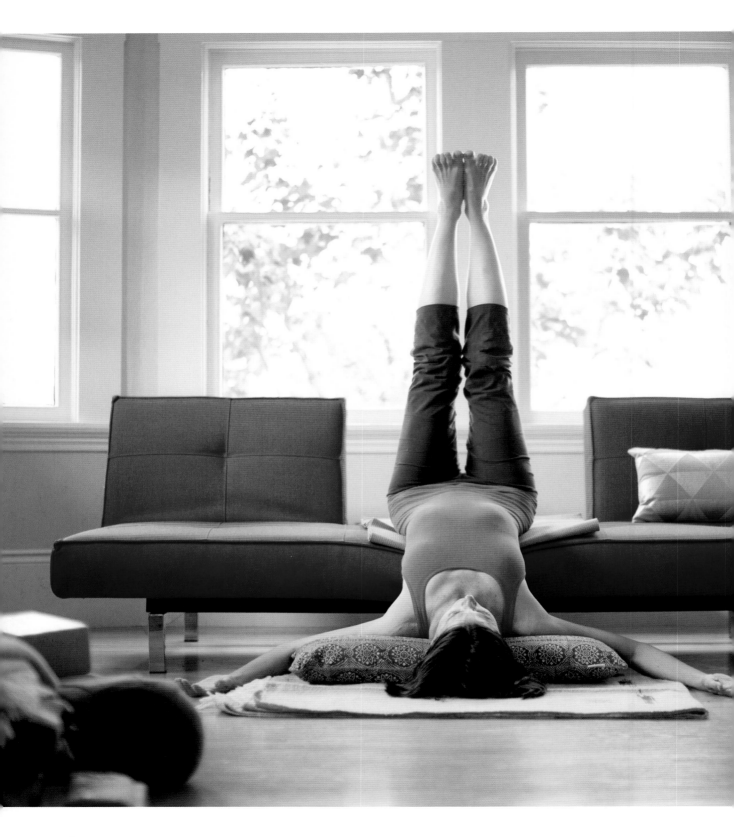

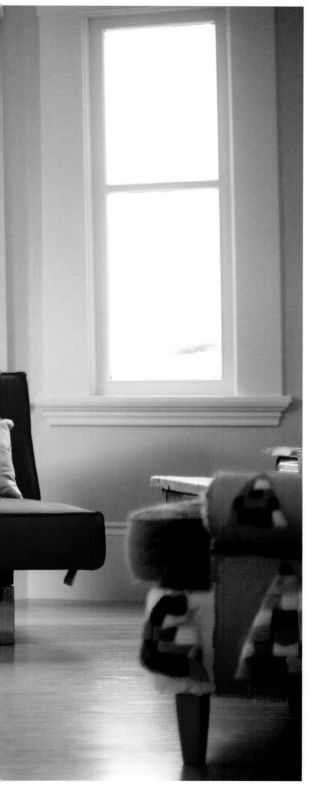

mat into action, I quickly jot them down. I usually end up with a list of phone calls to make, e-mails to write, and dust bunnies to destroy.

I try to do a 20-minute Savasana every day. That can happen on my mat or in my bed or in someone else's living room, but I practice the alignment of Savasana and I work with my breath and my mind. My practice also sometimes involves reading a spiritual text, or listening to an online dharma talk.

I let go of the "shoulds" of sequencing. I know oh so well how to sequence a class for others, but for myself I can put the rules aside. Wheel might be the second pose. I might come into Lotus without any hip openers or do Savasana in the middle of a sequence. I listen and let my body guide me. It's great fun when I can fully get out of my own way and let my body do the sequencing and teaching.

I now understand that my home practice happens off the mat as much as on. Can I let go of my agenda and listen to my husband and child? On the street, can I make eye contact with someone who appears to be suffering? Can I sprinkle in a little extra kindness to the barista making my beverage? Can I empty my own mind to be more present for my students? Can I remember to breathe deeply when life begins to feel like a tornado? Can I slow down and enjoy the journey instead of living in my habit to rush? I ask myself these types of questions every day.

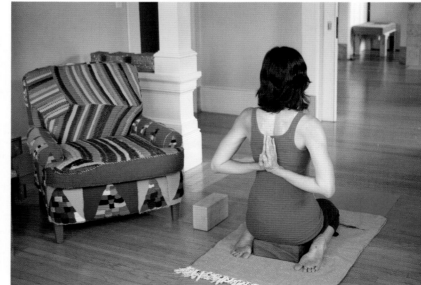

"Through meditation we connect most deeply with the sacred stillness inside the heart."

Sally Kempton

CARMEL VALLEY, CALIFORNIA | MEDITATION TEACHER/AUTHOR

A disciple of Swami Muktananda and the author of several books, Sally is one of America's most authentic spiritual teachers. She offers heart-to-heart transmission in meditation and life practice through her Awakening Heart workshops.

I can't imagine life without practice. I've been practicing meditation for about forty-five years, and I depend on my daily immersion in the inner witness, in nondual consciousness, and in devotional relationships with the deity. It has carried me through every personal crisis of these past years, from daily stress to illness to radical life changes. It is where I go for answers to questions, to chill out, to get help from within, and to simply enjoy the sacred self.

It is through meditation that we connect most deeply with the core of ourselves, the sacred stillness inside the heart. Meditation creates powerful, proven shifts in brain processes, helps develop an active witness, and, above all, opens us to the extraordinary

SALLY'S PRACTICE ADVICE

⚜ Use the space you have, make the practice as portable as possible, and, above all, create a habit. Surround your practice with beauty to make it attractive. Also have an altar if possible.

⚜ Don't feel that you have to do a full practice if your time is short. Even doing one asana or 10 minutes of meditation is better than no practice at all! Create a short practice, a medium practice, and a long practice so you can alternate depending on the time you have, and take brief asana or meditation breaks during the day.

⚜ Reading a spiritual book can also be a huge inspiration at the beginning and end of a practice.

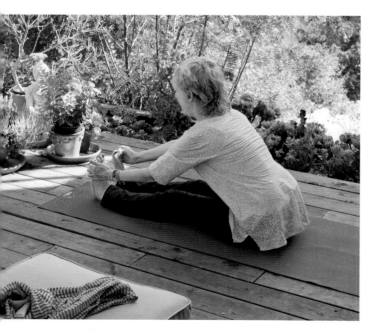

depths of wonder, love, and spontaneous wisdom that every human being holds within. Without meditation, we remain on the surface of ourselves. Daily meditation is an opportunity to check in regularly with the peace behind the mind, and, as you practice it, the mind becomes more focused, manageable, calm, and creative. And meditation can be practiced when our bodies won't allow us to practice asana—even when we're bedridden. You can meditate on an airplane or a bus, so it is an incredibly portable practice! This is especially true when meditation is combined with mantra and pranayama—even very simple pranayama.

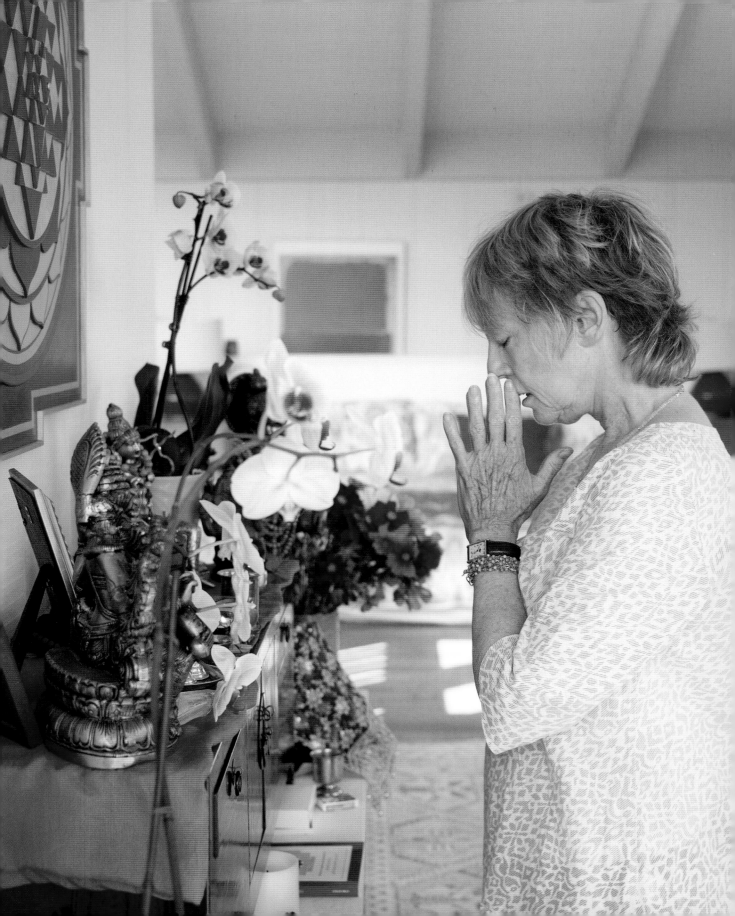

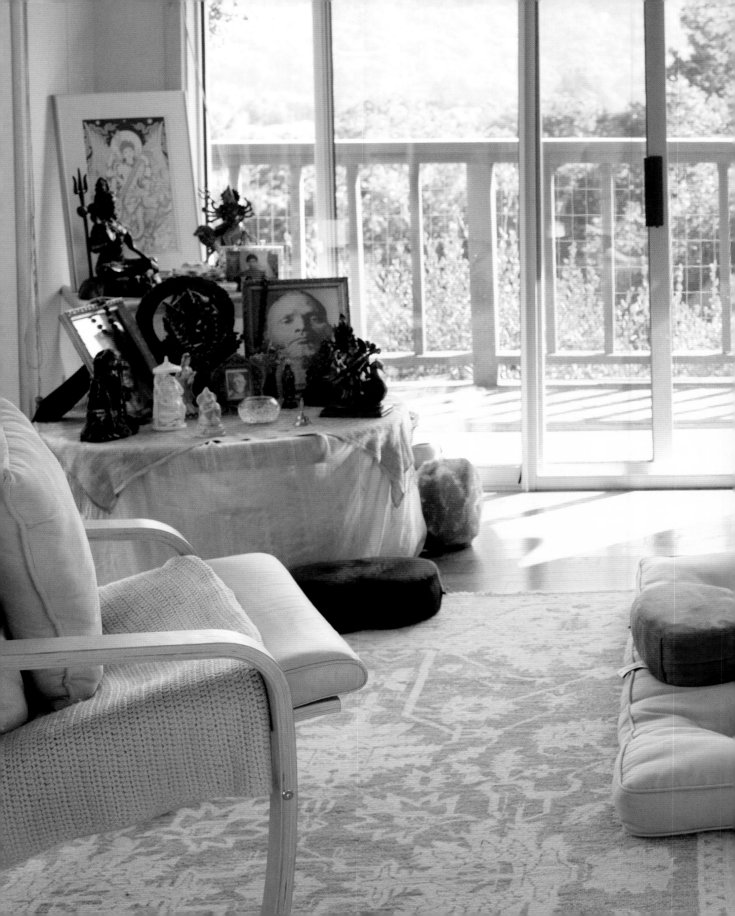

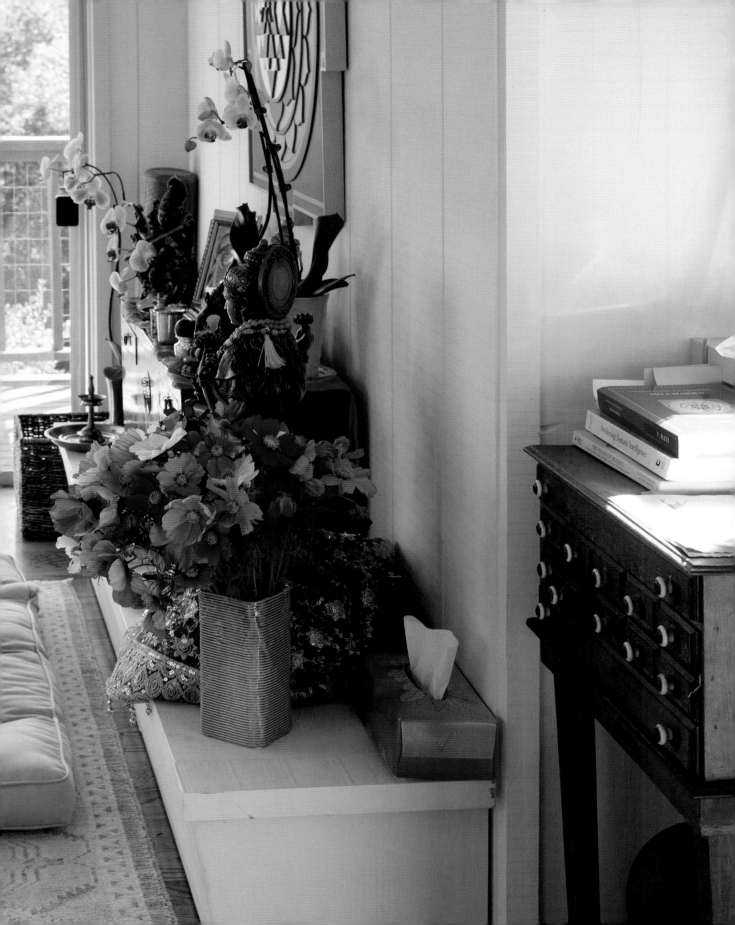

"I sensed myself venturing toward Spirit, and I felt that the practice was something sacred."

Rod Stryker

CARBONDALE, COLORADO | YOGA TEACHER

As founder of ParaYoga, Rod is a leading voice for the ancient traditions. His down-to-earth approach is informed as much by his mastery of the sublime teachings as it is by his love of life and devotion to his wife and four children.

Even though I began my personal practice nearly thirty-five years ago, I can still vividly recall the power of those first few sessions. I was just a fledgling, but I felt as though I was staking out precious space and time as the world outside—the traffic below my window included—continued its noisy march. I sensed myself venturing toward Spirit, and although it would take a while before any devout experiences dawned, I felt that the practice itself was something sacred. I saw it as walking into life's greatest challenge, one that was hands down the most rewarding of all— self-knowledge. After only a day or two, I was hooked.

I had found a companion for life. Nothing I gleaned from my studies in philosophy and psychology in college could equal the peace and inspiration that I was experiencing.

Over the years, there have been very few interruptions in what became a daily practice. I am often asked how I manage to practice every day; I have taught and met thousands who say they want to practice as well, but for whatever reason they find it hard or impossible to do. The simple answer is I quickly learned how much of a difference it made when I practiced, and how I just did not want to go through a day without the

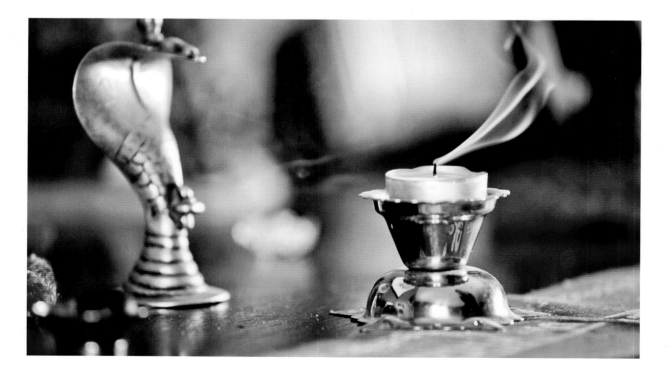

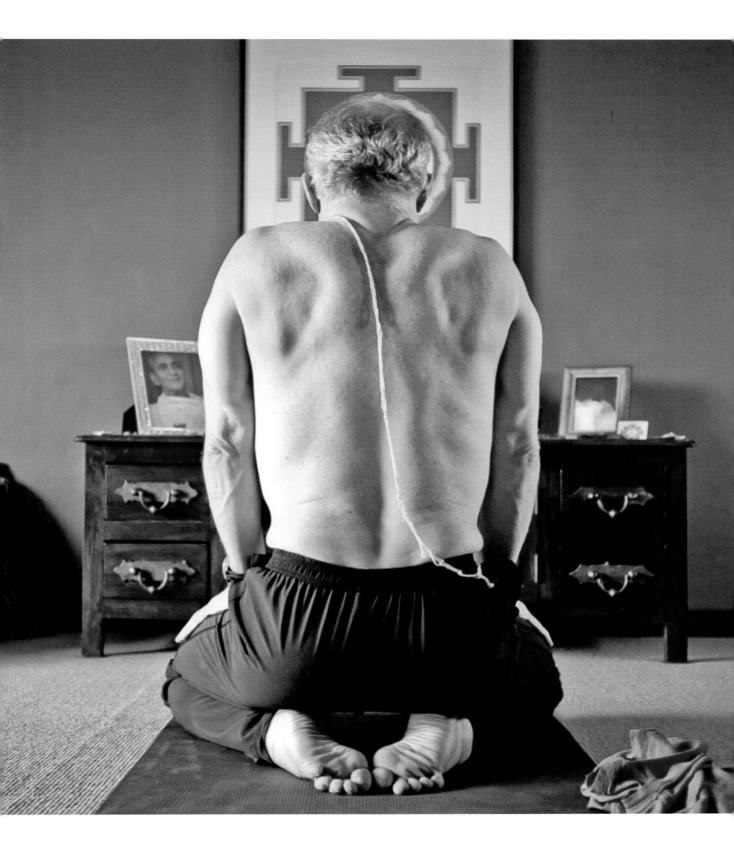

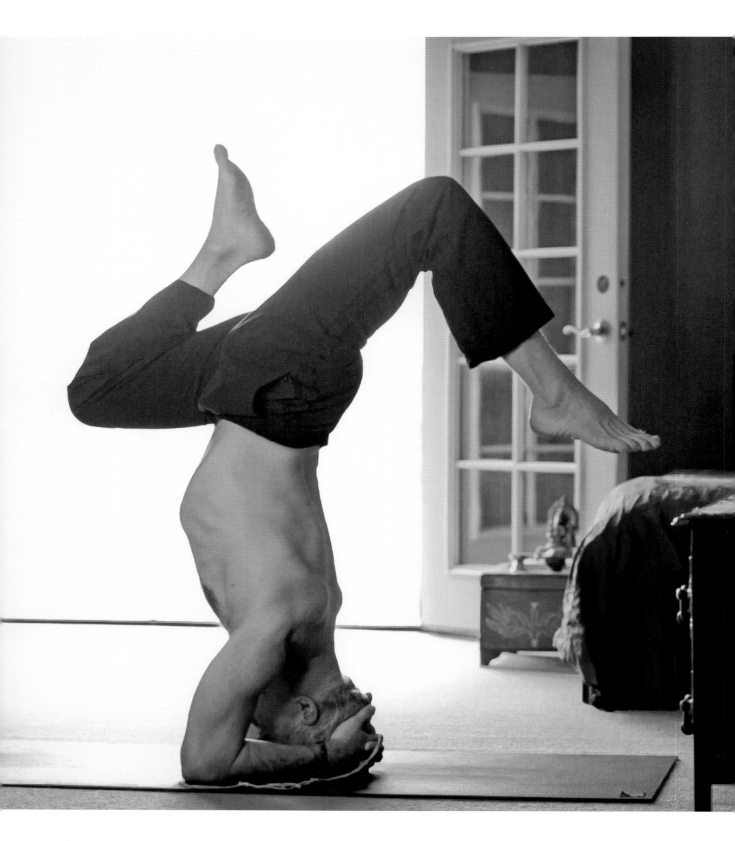

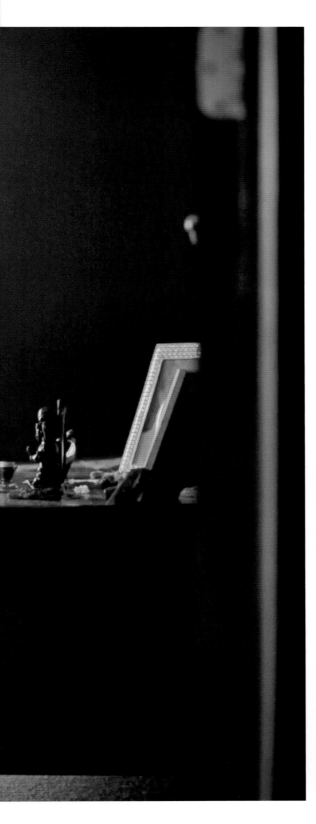

benefits that practice provided. At a deeper level, there was this abiding sense that I would only become the I was meant to be if I practiced every day; the only way I could navigate my way to the life I truly wanted was to consistently settle into the version of me that only practice could reveal.

My practice has always lasted somewhere between 1½ to 3 hours, with at least half of that time devoted to meditation. As far as what I practice, I am fairly unique. I have always had a teacher, a master, who has prescribed a personal meditation practice for me. Old school. That's how I became a yogi. But for asana and pranayama, I simply draw on my decades of teaching for inspiration. I've experimented and learned over the years, always adjusting this part of my practice to help me meet the demands of life and my changing needs. Some days that means a more energetically powerful practice; sometimes a more nurturing or steadying one would be more beneficial. My aim is to ensure the most meaningful and rich meditation practice possible. Meditation has always been my focus; I'm quite certain it always will be.

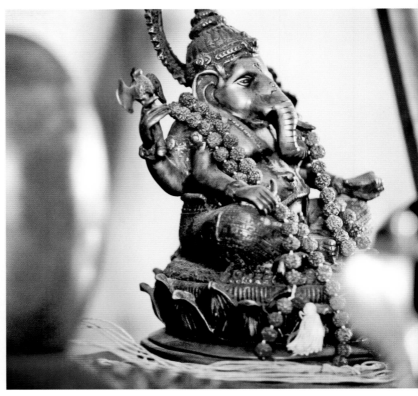

"I feel that my soul is fed through the practice of meditation and yoga."

Mey Elbi

ISTANBUL, TURKEY | YOGA TEACHER

Since returning to her home country from New York, where she trained in OM yoga, Mey has become one of Istanbul's leading yoga teachers and loves to share her experience and understanding of this ancient awareness practice.

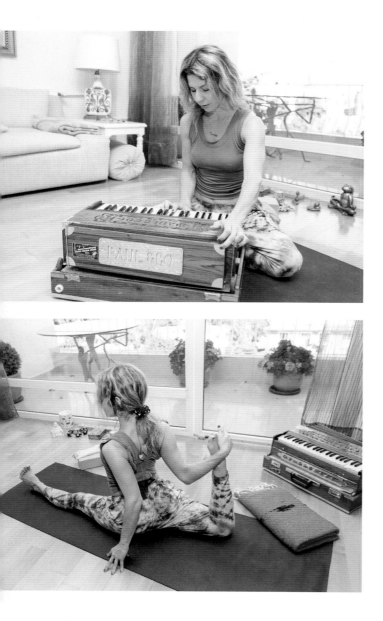

I love the light and the view from my place. It looks out onto the beautiful Bosphorus in Istanbul. Seen from up the hill, the sea and the sky make me happy. My favorite spot in my new home is the living room, where I feel connected to the open space.

I have little pieces that remind me of my connection to the Divine, such as Ganesha and some Buddha sculptures, and I am surrounded by lots of yoga books. With incense and some candles, I create the space.

When I practice by myself, I can go deeper into what I need and feel. That gives me a sense of deep listening and intimacy. Yoga is about listening and hearing, looking and seeing. Yoga is an inquiry into our darkness and shadows so that we can light them up slowly. Yoga helps me to find inner joy, peace, and my full potential. I become more and more at ease with who I am, where I am.

In my home practice I listen to my body. I follow my body's sensations, needs, and intuition to flow. Meditation and pranayama are the key elements of

MEY'S PRACTICE ADVICE

- Your practice doesn't have to only be asana based. Listening to music, dancing, and meditation help me to ground, energize, and dive deeper. And being alone, in contemplation or in reading yoga-related books—that's yoga, too.

- Just get a mat. Be on your mat. And remember: you can do yoga anywhere.

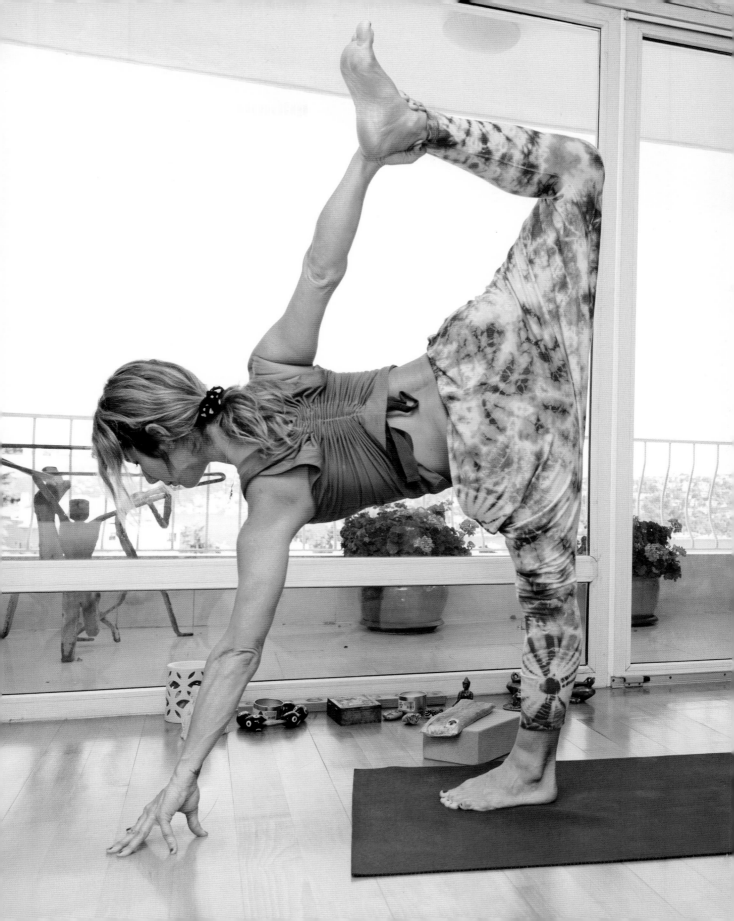

MEY'S SAMPLE PRACTICE

- Sit in meditation for 5 minutes

- Nadi Shodhana Pranayama (Alternate Nostril Breathing) for 5 minutes

- Surya Namaskar (Sun Salutations) for 10 minutes

- Any forward bending pose, such as Tarasana (Star Pose) or Paschimottanasana (Seated Forward Bend)

- Any seated twist, such as Bharadvajasana (Easy Twisting Pose)

- Any backbending pose, such as Setu Bandha Sarvangasana (Bridge Pose)

- Supta Baddha Konasana (Reclining Bound Angle Pose) for 5 minutes

- Savasana (Corpse Pose)

my practice. Through my practice, I have a more intimate connection with myself. I become centered and grounded. Observing my body, feelings, and thoughts from a distance allows me to create a healthy relationship with my physical, emotional, and mental body. That expanded awareness is what gives the healing. To awaken to the present moment is what gives me the connection and joy. And to encounter my fear, my weakness, and my obstacles gives me inner strength. I feel that my soul is fed through the practice of meditation and yoga.

My yoga practice is not limited to the mat. Everything inspires me—a wise sentence, a nice piece of music, a smile, a tear, a fear. Yoga is about feeling, about being in touch with our humanly part. Of course, there will always be distractions. It is good to include these distractions in your practice as well. See your reactions to it. If there are no obstacles, your journey did not start. Despite the challenges in and out, can you go deeper? That is my search.

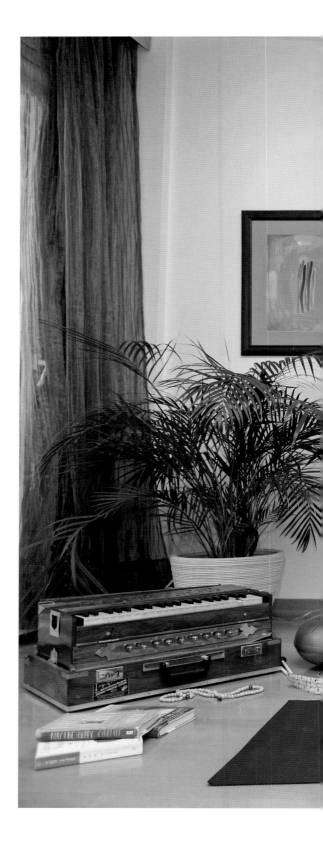

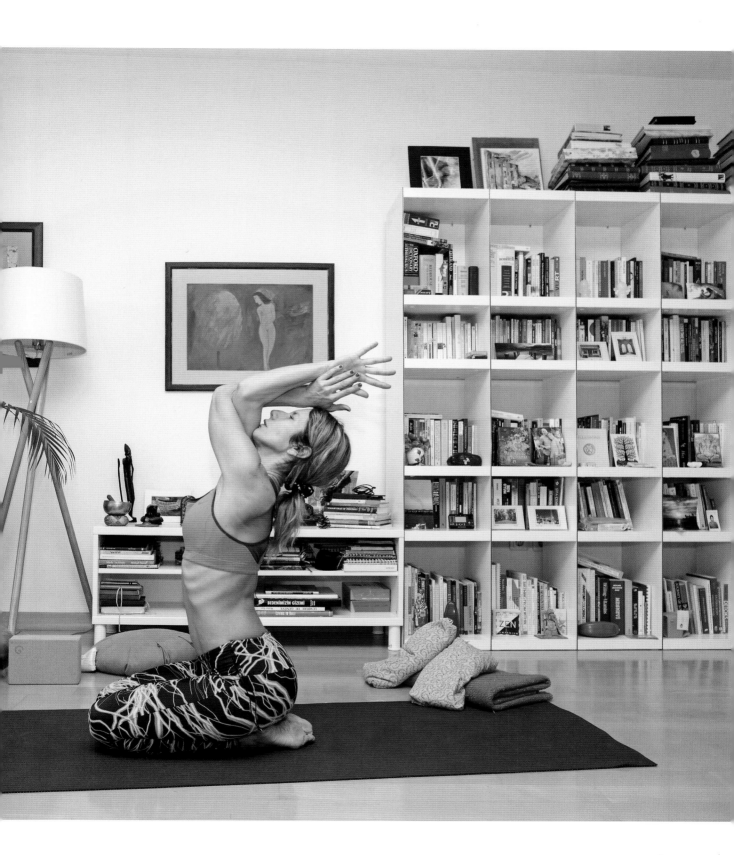

127

"My yoga space is the only clear place I have among all the stuff in my house."

Isaac Mukwaya

NAIROBI, KENYA | YOGA TEACHER

Isaac's love of music and dance infuses his Baptiste yoga practice. An Africa Yoga Project teacher, Isaac honors his own teachers, Baron Baptiste and Paige Elenson, and continues to learn from them.

My yoga space is the only clear place I have among all the stuff in my house. I usually play music while I practice, and the connection to the music there is easy. What to practice just comes to me. But sometimes the warm-up takes longer than other times. I do aerobic kinds of exercises and some dance moves that I learned from a fellow yoga teacher, Cheloti, to heat up the body. My desire to learn Handstand also inspires me to practice.

ISAAC'S PRACTICE ADVICE

- Work on self-discipline, cultivate passion, and be eager to grow.
- Baron Baptiste says that a good teacher has a good practice and from that practice you become a bad-ass teacher.

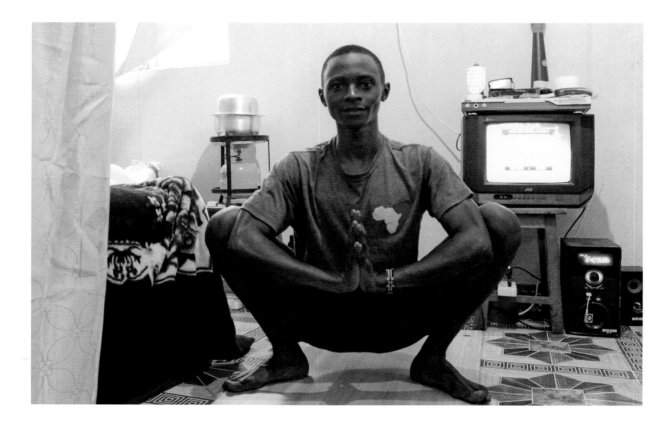

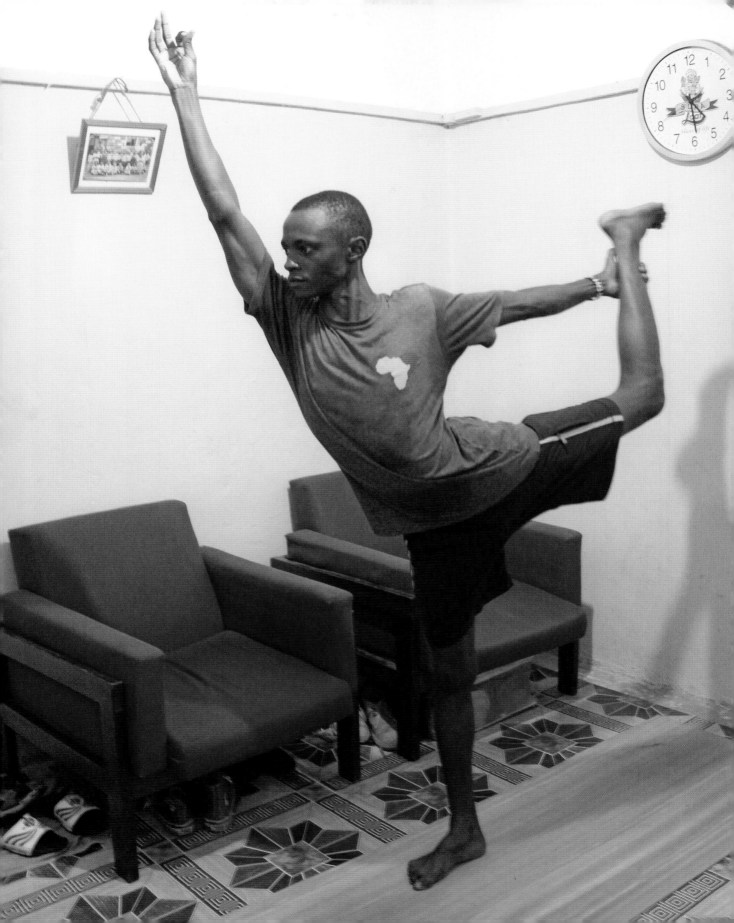

"One of the greatest things about practicing at home is that I get to be alone."

Linnea Vedder

NEW YORK, NEW YORK | YOGA TEACHER/ARTIST

As a Kripalu yoga teacher, artist, and musician, Linnea creates a fun and loving space for practitioners to explore their practice, in which she integrates a strong foundation of alignment with a balance of heat-building vinyasa.

We lovingly refer to our apartment as the "Zen center" because of the calming and simple environment we have created with white walls, plants, a few pieces of art, and small altars around the space. When I meditate, I can just grab a pillow from the sofa and blast off.

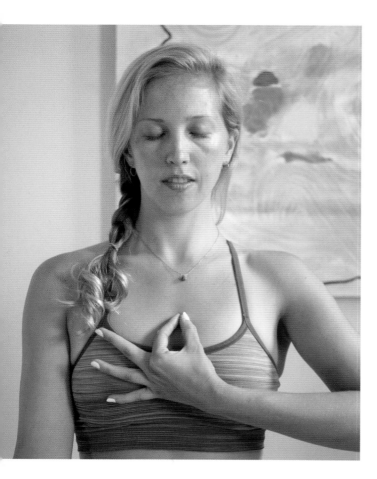

Creating sacred space means having a silent place to practice, putting my phone away, closing my eyes, breathing, and withdrawing my senses. One of the greatest things about practicing at home is that I get to be alone, which sometimes feels like the Holy Grail after a day in New York being squeezed into a subway car with hundreds of other human sardines. If it's not too hot in my apartment, I close the windows to shut out the noise from the street. If my partner is at home, I will sometimes close the French doors to create a private space where I can explore my practice more deeply and soak up what it feels like to live in my unique body.

My yoga practice has been a backbone of my life since I was a teenager. Almost five years ago, I became a yoga teacher and around that time I started

LINNEA'S PRACTICE ADVICE

❁ It can feel weird, silly, or confusing to practice without a teacher, but if you just "fake it 'til you make it" at the beginning, you'll soon be doing it for real. Getting to know your *satguru*, or inner teacher, takes time, so be patient with yourself. It's OK to copy other people. Take notes on what you like in a class or look online for inspiration.

❁ Have fun! Allow yourself to loosen up by making weird noises and allowing your body to guide you into strange positions.

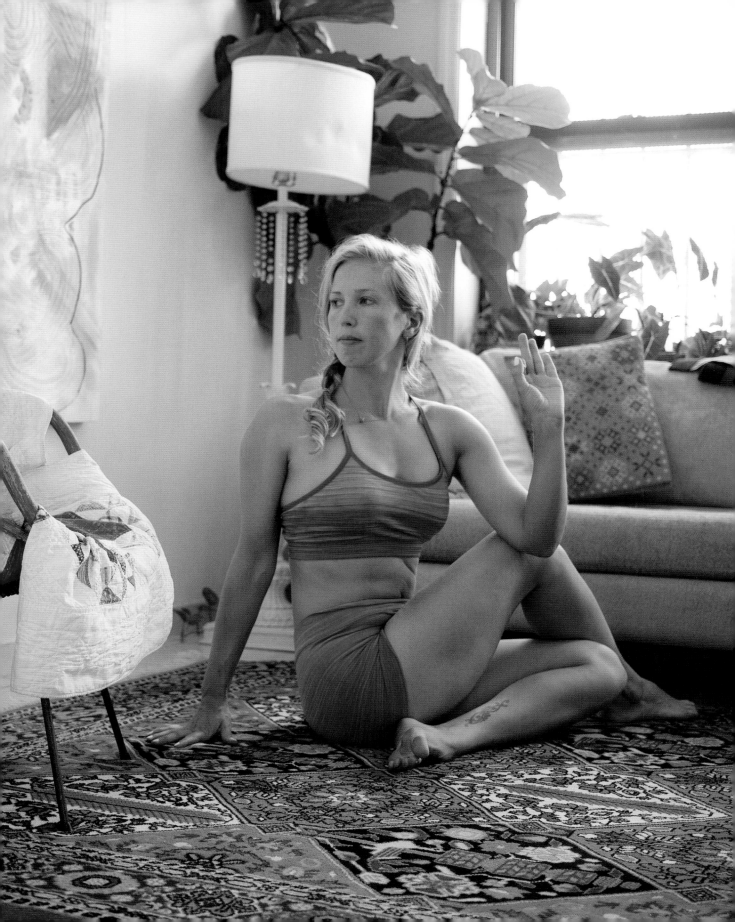

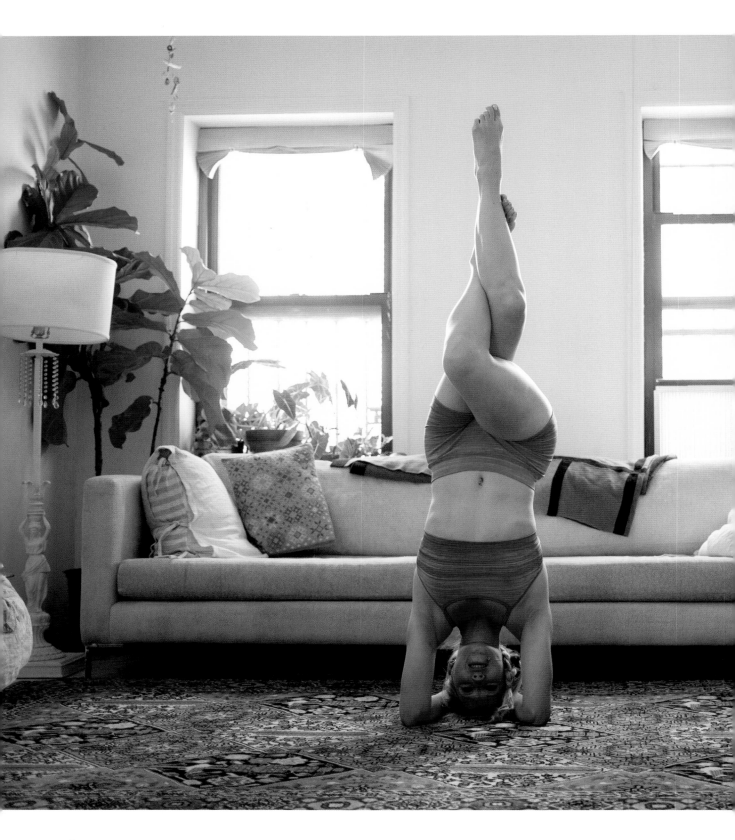

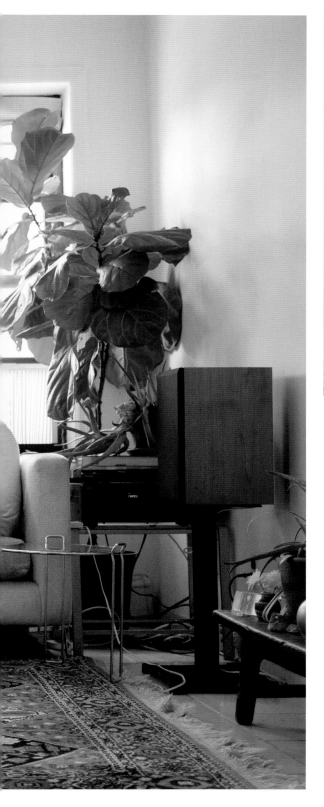

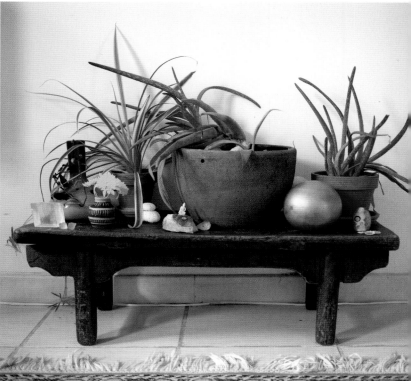

to practice at home more diligently. The process of becoming a teacher helped me to overcome my shyness, while the practice of doing yoga by myself taught me quite literally how to take up space. I learned that I was afraid to take up space energetically and I didn't feel worthy of asking to have my own space. Through practicing alone, I was able to become more myself and more empowered to do my karmic work of painting, teaching, and loving.

Taking yoga on the road served me when I was a traveling musician and it now helps me stay focused when I paint. I don't even need a mat or any props at my studio; I simply step onto the wood floor. It's very freeing to not be beholden to a gym or equipment and to be free to practice wherever I have enough space to stretch out my arms. I do a short meditation before I paint, which helps me focus and ground my art practice.

> *"Home practice is like home cooking; you can't get it anywhere else and there's nothing quite like it."*

Giselle Mari

MENLO PARK, CALIFORNIA | YOGA TEACHER

Known for her dynamic Jivamukti classes, Giselle fuses funky music, chanting, skillful hands-on assists, an insightful topic for mind, body, and spirit, and an asana practice that will light your fire and send you home glowing.

Asana means seat, or connection to the earth and all its beings. You may not have the option to experience your Downward-Facing Dog, forward bend, or backbend every single day, but you always have an opportunity to open yourself up to a different point of view, bow in reverence to another being, or bend over backward for someone in need. Anytime you have a chance to create peace for others or inspire them to be

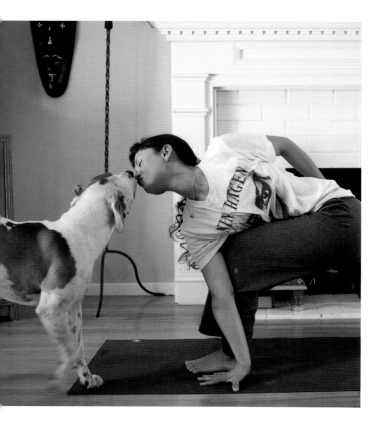

their best by your actions of kindness, whether that is physically, mentally, spiritually, or energetically, you are practicing yoga asana.

Every room in my home has some reminder of my spiritual practice, whether it's a picture, a *murti* (an image of a god or goddess), or my altar. It's not only a mental reminder, but also an energetic charge for my living space and everyone who enters into it. So although I feel I can practice anywhere in my house, I love practicing in my living room. My altar is there, as well as my bay window that looks out to the backyard. I may be practicing inside, but I feel very connected to the serenity of the outdoors and I get to experience the seasonal changes as well—which in California is only two seasons.

My home practice starts just after I wake up. I sit up in bed and begin my silent *japa* (mantra). I let the mantra come to me; if it doesn't appear, I'll chant one that was given to me by my teachers. I do one round on my mala beads, at which point I set an intention for my day. From there, I go to my altar and meditate somewhere between 5 and 30 minutes, and follow it up with an asana practice for 15 to 90 minutes, depending on what my schedule looks like for that day.

Anytime I move into practicing yoga, whether I practice asana, meditation, pranayama, or all of the above, the space morphs to my energy and intention, so it's not like I have to delineate the space. I just make it so. It's all about perspective. One moment it's my living room with a television and a fireplace; another moment it becomes a sweet space for my spiritual practice; and then it's a space for hanging out with my family and dogs. It is all sacred, all the time.

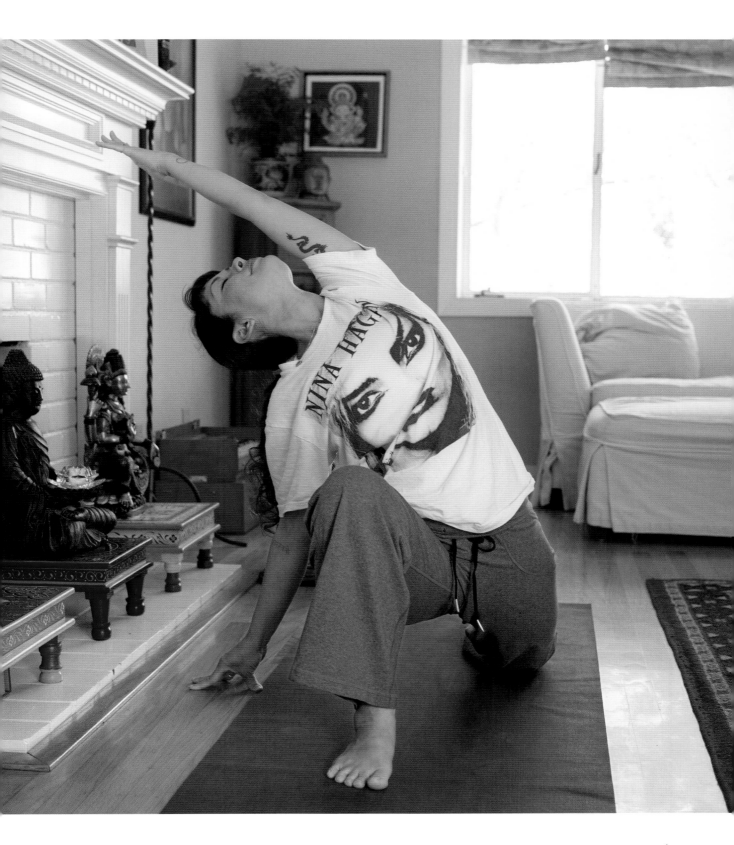

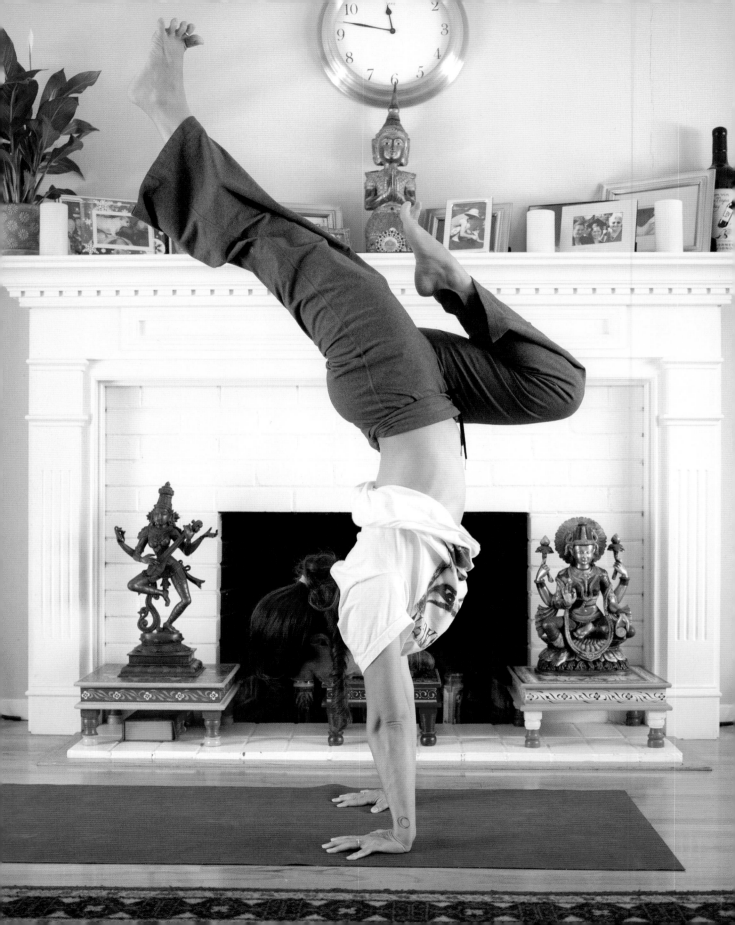

GISELLE'S PRACTICE ADVICE

〜 Home practice is like home cooking; you can't get it anywhere else and there's nothing quite like it. You can experiment and break the "rules." Play music or don't play music. Shelve the stretchy pants and wear those old sweats and a T-shirt. Explore poses that really speak to you, poses you have little relationship with but are curious about, and of course even dance with the ones you don't like. Each asana is an ingredient in the yoga recipe for your soul. What do you want to create and feed yourself with? The options are endless and are only limited by your imagination.

〜 Since the hardest part is starting, hook your soul up and do a little preplanning to ensure your practice happens. Lay out all your yoga gear the night before so it's one less thing you have to set up. Let's face it—something as small as having to locate your mat or blocks can easily become the obstacle that lures you back to the couch, answering e-mails, or emptying out your dishwasher.

〜 Start slow, keep it simple, and be consistent. Do a once-a-week practice that includes a series of gentle movements or basic Sun Salutations and a 5-minute meditation; borrow a sequence from your teacher or another seasoned practitioner.

〜 Once you start, you may be encouraged to move more and stay longer. But don't beat yourself up or think you're a spiritual loser if you fall short or don't stay on your schedule. It is a practice after all, so start up again.

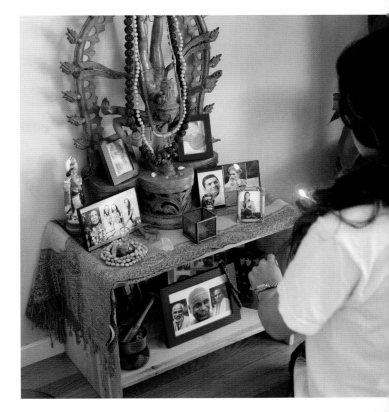

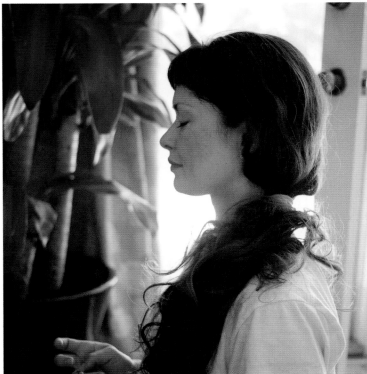

"Getting on the mat without an agenda is the key;
I surrender to what is arising from within."

Shibana Singh

SANTA FE, NEW MEXICO | YOGA TEACHER/AYURVEDIC PRACTITIONER

Shibana brings a wealth of knowledge, spirituality, and passion to her work in nutrition, ayurveda, yoga, and life coaching. She is known among her clients for her loving and holistic approach, no matter what their goals are.

My home practice is my prayer. I practice all over the house: in the living room and in the bedroom where I have my altars set up. My favorite place to practice is the living room with mantra

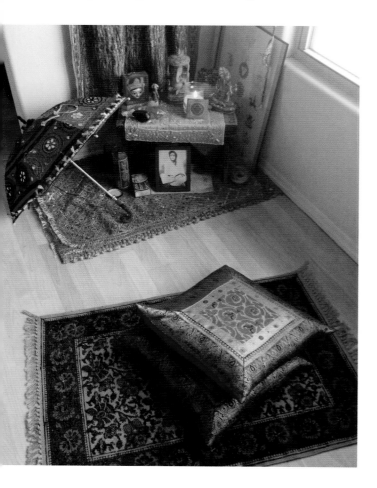

SHIBANA'S PRACTICE ADVICE

- Make your practice a discipline, a *sadhana*, until it becomes part of you, part of the body.

- Don't set difficult goals, but do whatever your calling may be on each day.

- Your practice doesn't have to be asana based. Asana is just one tool in the ultimate experience of *yogah chitta vritti nirodhah* (quieting the mind). Chanting, pranayama, conscious dance, and rituals—both spiritual and mundane—feed the soul. Those can all be part of your yoga practice, too.

playing in the background, the *deepak* (earthen oil lamp) lit in front of the altar and the beautiful energy of my daughter doing her work on the table while often glancing my way. Every space is sacred in my heart. The moment I unroll the mat and set my intentions the place becomes sacred.

Getting on the mat without an agenda is the key to my practice. If that means there will be days I will only be in Child's Pose, it is totally fine, because I surrender to what is arising from within, whether it is to dance the cosmic dance or to lie still. My practice has given me an anchor when everything outside was pulling me into the darkest of storms.

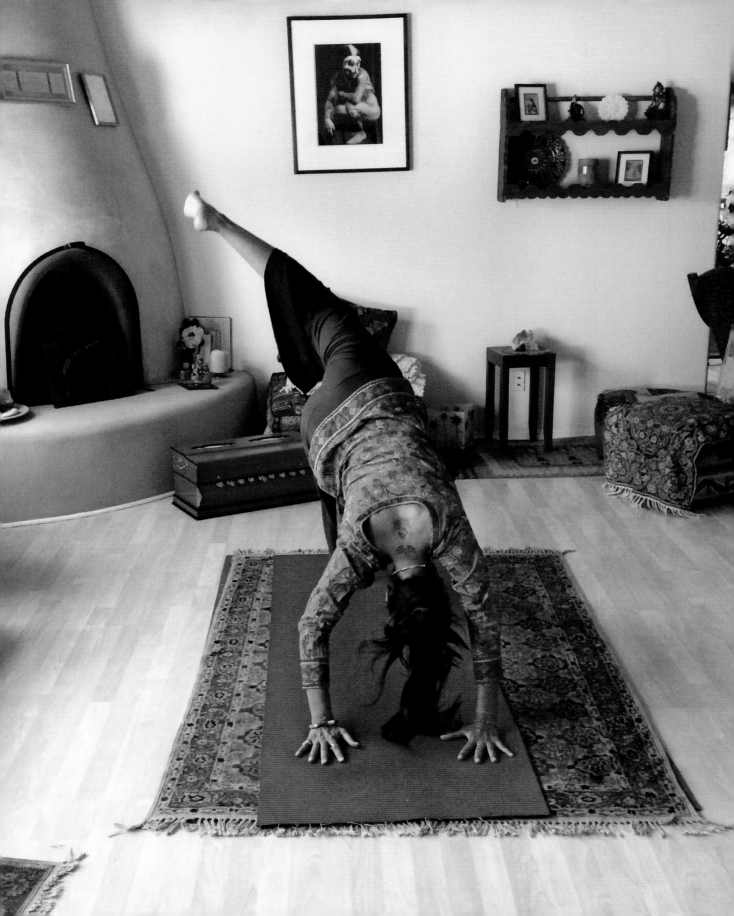

"When you're actively engaged in a heart-based practice, peace and love are inevitable."

Pan Trinity Das & Kyrie Maezumi

THE ROAD, UNITED STATES OF AMERICA | BHAKTI POP! ARTIST • DESIGNER/MUSICIAN

Bhakti POP! artist Pan paints street murals and designs bhakti-themed installations for festivals. He and Kyrie—designer, musician, and daughter of Zen Master Maezumi Roshi—are currently traveling the country in an RV.

We experience simplicity as sacred. It's a joy to have our favorite things be our only things, each having a story, beauty, and reminder. The entire RV has become a bit of an altar. Practice is what our lives revolve around now. And by practice, we do mean asanas but also clear communication, self-reflection, and having time to read and talk about ideas and growth. It feels a bit like a pilgrimage.

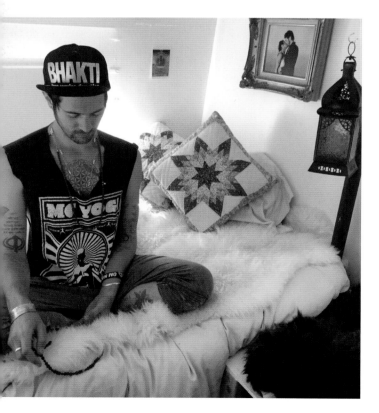

PAN: In an RV, your sacred space is with you one hundred percent of the time—something that I find helpful in remaining in a relaxed and positive state. My own personal sanctuary is available whether I'm running errands or stuck in traffic; it allows me to take refuge from the world and drop into what's really important—health and happiness. Another advantage of having an RV is all the many wonderful and sometimes random places you can take your practice. It always adds an exciting element of fun and adventure!

KYRIE: Living on the road has definitely changed the way I define home and family. There is very little separation in our lives between home and practice. We have to be mindful, conscientious of each other, attentive to our own self-care, and make sure that the space stays organized and clean.

PAN: For me, beauty brings inspiration and serenity. What I find to be beautiful just happens to be transcendent art, so that is what I surround myself with. I think it was Yogi Bhajan who said, "The only thing we are attracted to is sacredness."

KYRIE: We create sacred space with love and respect. I feel like the experience of sacred space is connection and presence. It can be with anything. A loved one, a rock, a candle flame, the action you take in the world.

PAN: I spend countless hours in nonjudgmental self-reflection. In my experience, keeping my body occupied with practice allows my mind to sift through transgressions and come to a place of inward resolution

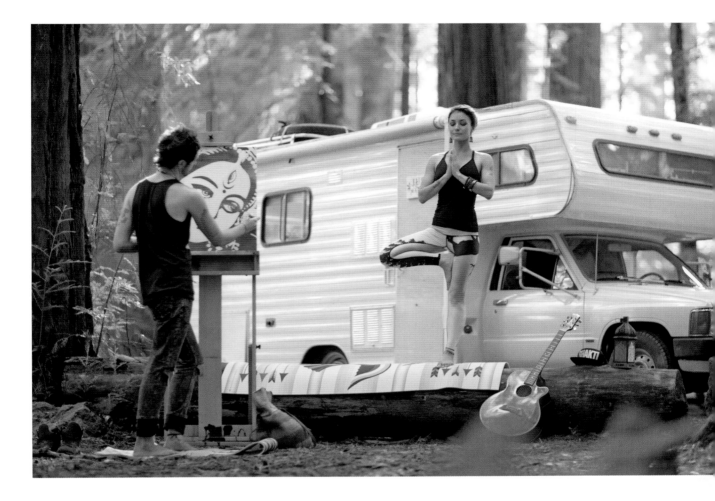

and hopefully wisdom. When you're actively engaged in a heart-based practice, peace and love are inevitable.

KYRIE: For me, practice is synonymous with patience. That is the space I cultivate and try to maintain. It is patience with myself most of all. It's so true that much suffering is caused by expectations; for me, it is health issues. I have a chronic back injury from a car accident and, being a dancer for most of my life, I've learned to listen to my body and check my ego when I want to be able to do what I used to be able to do. Every day is different; yoga is the constant and we are the variable. For me, it has been a journey of self-love and self-reflection, no goals, no attachment. Just the knowledge that when I make the time to breathe, bring attention to the blockages and tension that cause pain, and gently let go, my day is different, my body is happy. I feel gratitude.

PAN & KYRIE'S PRACTICE ADVICE

- Bhagavan Das has said that you should turn what you already love into your practice and we think that's great advice. If you enjoy cooking, make the main ingredient love. If you love money, make conscious investments. Offering your efforts to the Divine is not only the essence of bhakti, but also a platform for humanitarianism.

- Really listen to your body and get to know what will benefit you most. Take time to explore. It's essential that everyone define their own practice if they are going to carry it into their own daily lives.

"The act of standing on the mat itself provides the invitation to drop inside."

Kaitlin Quistgaard

MILL VALLEY, CALIFORNIA | PUBLISHING CONSULTANT/WRITER

Former editor in chief of *Yoga Journal*, Kaitlin creates products and services that inspire us all to make healthier choices. An avid bicyclist and world traveler, she is rarely separated from her practice.

I don't make a big effort to create sacred space. I unfurl my mat, breathe, and go. I used to have a dedicated practice space beside an altar, and I do know the lovely gravitational pull that can exert—the space itself offers an invitation to drop deeper; sometimes simply stepping into it shifts your awareness. But I've traded that for something less magical and more pragmatic: an integrated experience, where stepping onto my mat does not require any special force fields.

I do occasionally pull one of my deity statues down from the top shelf they migrated to after I disassembled my altar, especially if I'm in some phase of soul searching or longing for answers that I can't find with my rational mind. I sometimes enjoy reconnecting with the mystic elements!

But, mostly, I use my heart and mind to create whatever qualities I need for practice. I now see my mat as the container for my practice. The act of standing on the mat itself provides the invitation to drop inside.

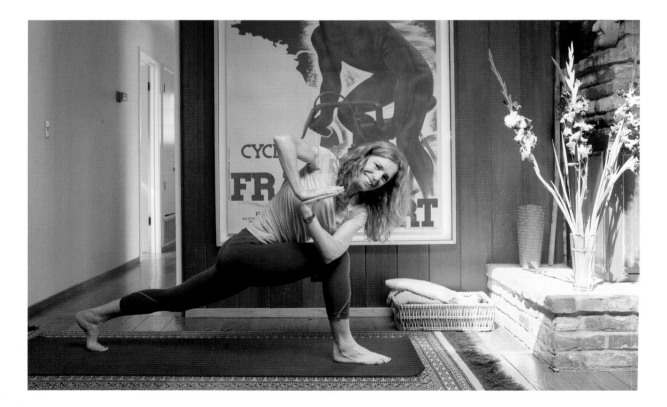

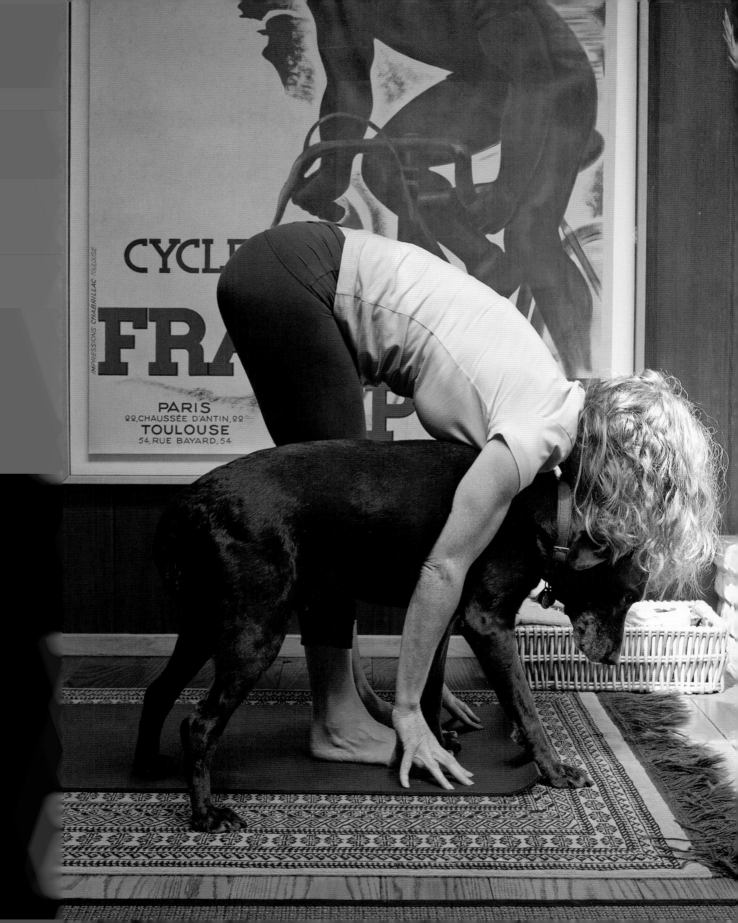

"I cherish my solo practice because it bathes me in a fountain of healing energy."

Sianna Sherman

LOS ANGELES, CALIFORNIA | YOGA TEACHER

Sianna weaves together traditional and contemporary wisdom in her multifaceted approach, which includes hatha yoga, vinyasa, Tantra, therapeutics, mythology, mantra, meditation, and the power of practice for everyday transformation.

My personal practice is the source of my strength, endurance, patience, courage, tenacity, and willingness to be transparent and vulnerable. Through *sadhana* (spiritual practice), I establish my most intimate connection with the universal field of love. There are so many ways to invoke Spirit in our lives, so many paths of direct inner truth, and so many

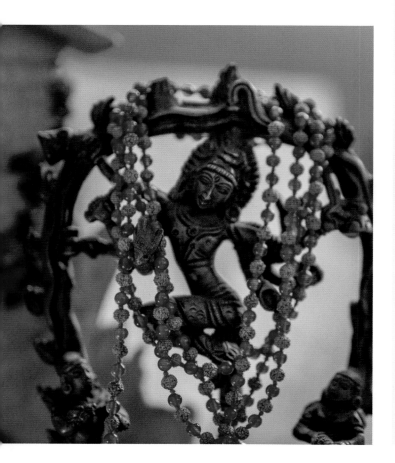

SIANNA'S PRACTICE ADVICE

◊ Set up the basic rhythm of your day to include sadhana. Early morning is very nice to set the tone of the day, but not everyone can practice in the early morning. If your time is limited, go stand outside with your feet on the earth, breathe deeply, and gaze upon the rising sun for a few minutes to energize yourself. If you have children, you can practice in the late morning once the kids are at school, in the afternoon, or even at night when everyone is sleeping. You choose! Look at the overall rhythm of the day and assess what works best for you in your daily flow.

◊ Regular practice over a long period of time is essential for the benefits of practice to ripen. In the yoga tradition, the Sanskrit word *abhyasa* means committed practice over a long period of time.

◊ Create a sadhana space that's inviting and beautiful to you. For some people, beauty is in simplicity and they thrive with a spacious environment with minimal colors or objects. Other practitioners resonate with multiple colors, altars, photos, and images of the Divine. The main thing is to listen within and create your space in a way that reflects your inner temple and calls you home to your practice.

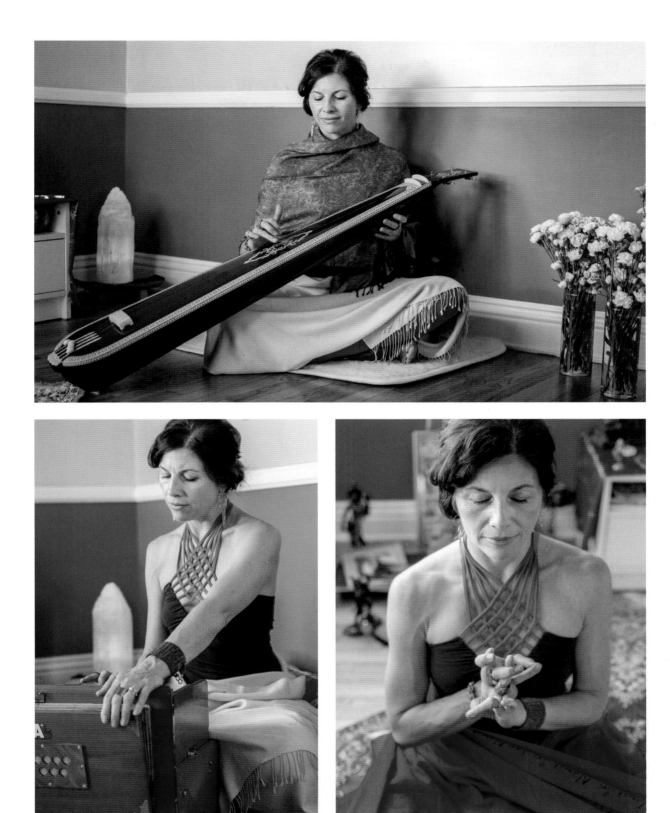

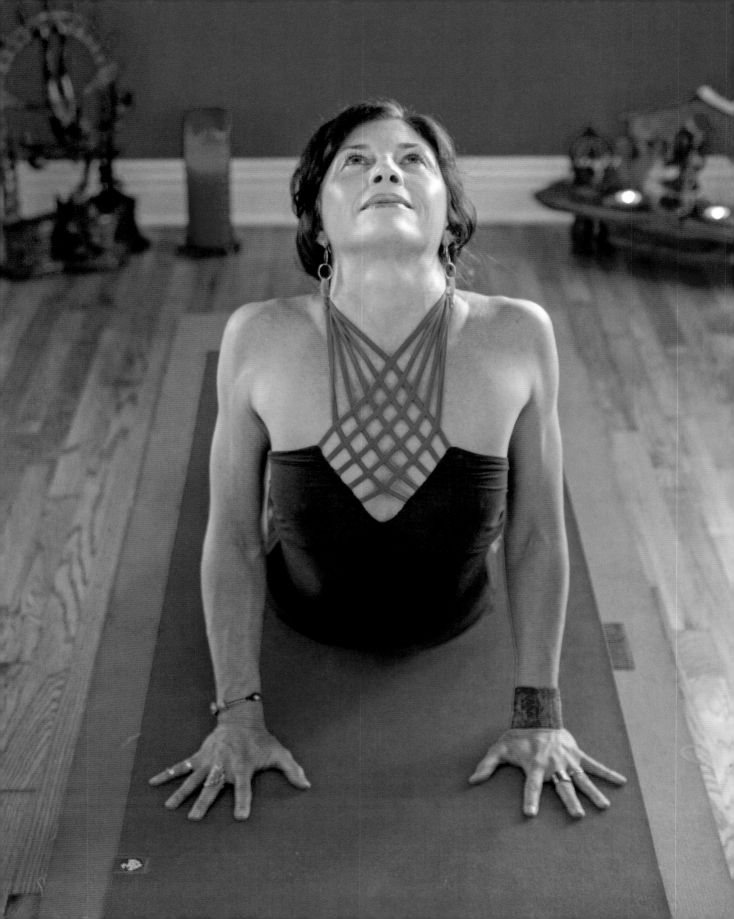

names we can call it: God, Goddess, Divine Mother, Consciousness, Great Void, Totality, Brahman, etc. Ultimately, it doesn't really matter what we call it. The most important thing is our direct experience of our own true nature, and for this we must courageously dive inside and do the work. For me, the way of direct experience is paved by my personal commitment to sadhana, prayer, and devotion.

I am a gypsy-hearted traveler and create sacred space wherever I land. I always set up a little area for my sadhana. It can be very simple: my prayer shawl, mantra rosary beads, and a flower. Sometimes I will connect inwardly to my physical home altar even from a distance. Some part of my altar will light up in my awareness and the connection is always there.

I cherish my solo practice because it bathes me in a fountain of rejuvenation and healing energy. I highly encourage all my students to establish a solo sadhana in addition to practicing in community gatherings.

Home practice helps us all experience an inner steadiness; greater adaptability in life; spaciousness within for listening to our truth; remembrance of what really matters; healthy integration of body, mind, heart, and soul; and ultimately the highest connection with the inner Divine Beloved.

SIANNA'S SAMPLE PRACTICE

- Choose a form of the Divine that resonates with you. This can be whatever speaks to you: a flower, photo of a teacher, a flame, an image of a deity, or even a blank canvas.

- Sit with your eyes softly open. Rest your awareness in the flow of your breath. Gaze softly upon the object in front of you, yet rest your inner gaze on the root of your heart.

- Allow the outer form to teach you about yourself. It is a reflection of you.

- After a few minutes, gently close your eyes and rest in the natural flow of your breath.

- Chant this beautiful mantra softly to yourself for several minutes: "*Aham prema*," which means "I am divine love."

- Continue to sit for some time, dwelling in the inner luminous field that is you.

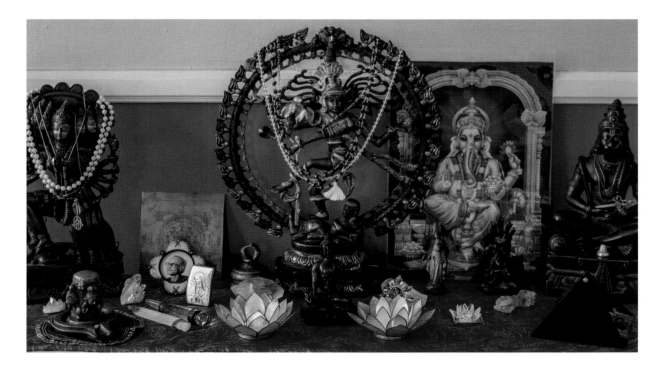

"When we are awake and caffeinated, it's prayer and meditation time."

Jan Schmidt & Arthur Rivers

NEW YORK, NEW YORK | CURATOR • RETIRED HAIRDRESSER

Curator of the Jerome Robbins Dance Division/New York City Public Library for the Performing Arts, Jan and her husband, Arthur, a retired hairdresser, practice together in their tiny apartment in New York City's East Village.

We've been together for twenty-six years. We started doing meditation as part of the practice of living a clean and sober life. Around the same time, Jan began to do yoga and African dance, which together are a great workout. She read an article about a test they did with the army or something, which said that 12 minutes a day of meditation made a statistical difference. So that's when we started timing ourselves. Our daily practice actually begins with feeding the cats, getting coffee, and sitting in bed checking e-mail. Then, when we are awake, caffeinated, and have had our fill of social media, it's prayer and meditation time.

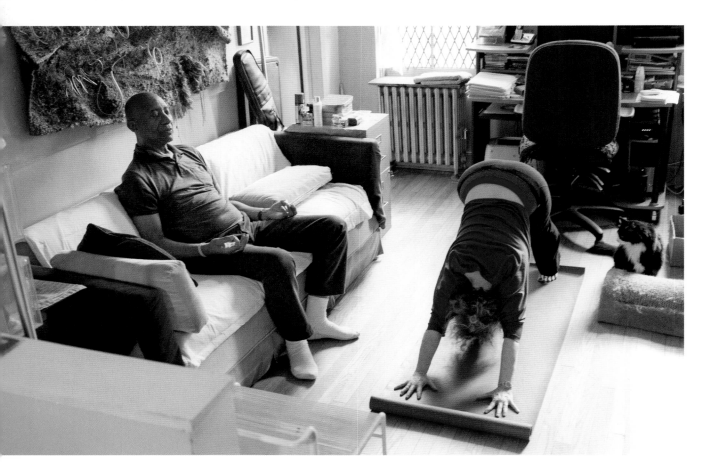

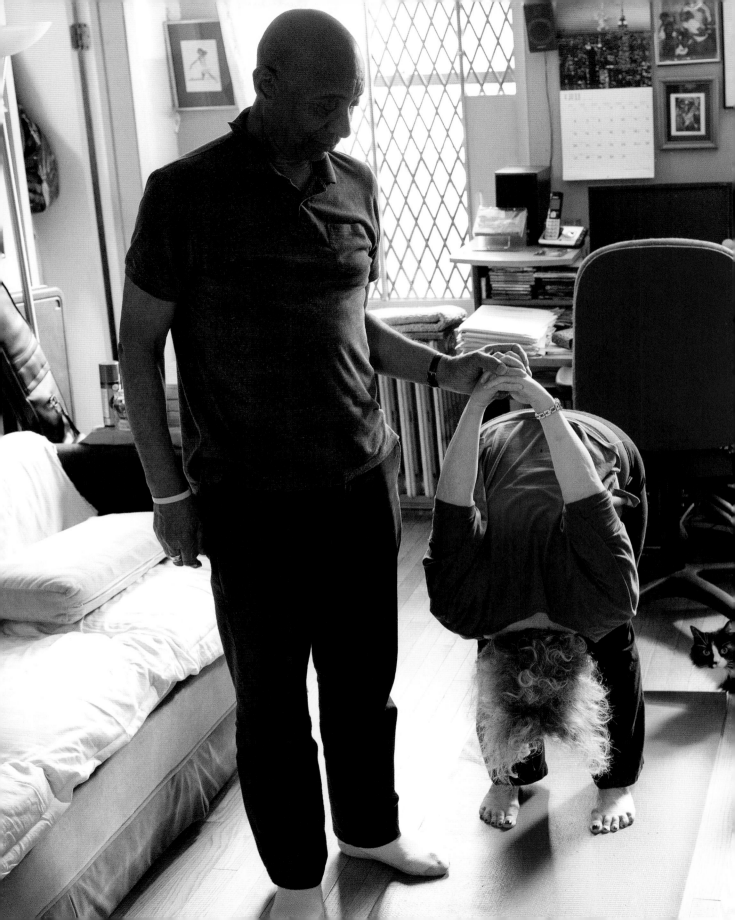

> *"I think the perfect place to practice is right here. The perfect time is right now."*

Miko Matsumura

LOS GATOS, CALIFORNIA | CHIEF MARKETING OFFICER, GRADLE

Deeply immersed in the ancient teachings of the *Bhagavad Gita* and the *Yoga Sutra*, Miko by day is a Silicon Valley executive who readily admits to applying the *Gita*'s philosophy of love to his work in "start-up land."

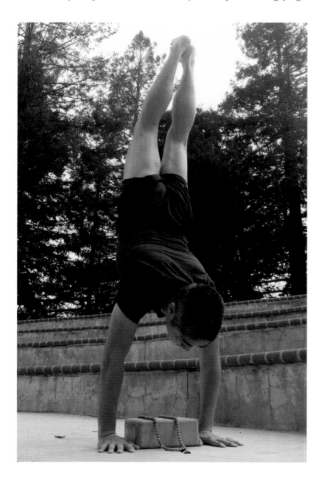

The *Hatha Yoga Pradipika* says your home practice should be somewhere that is "neither too low nor too high." But what if you don't have a choice in where you practice? What if you're practicing yoga on an airplane? Is that "too high?" To sustain a daily practice I often must practice wherever I find myself: in hotels, airports, parks, work, boats, and, yes, on airplanes. So, I make my yoga block my "home." Why do I even need a block? In part, just to have a devotional object that represents my practice. But at the heart of my home practice are seated poses and the block supports my sitting bones so my legs don't fall asleep. It's neither too soft nor too hard. Of course, the *Hatha Yoga Pradipika* also says you need a four-square-cubit room in a country where justice is properly administered. But do you know what I think? I think the perfect place to practice is right here. The perfect time is right now. Even if it's not perfect, it's perfect.

When I first started practicing, I set up a properly sacred-looking meditation space in my room with an altar and cushion—the works. One day, I took my block and went out to the garden to meditate. To my surprise, it was just as holy out there as it was in front of my altar. After that I started behaving as a cat does, each day choosing my seat in a picky, yet seemingly random, way. Once this became established, my block became the only constant in my everyday practice and eventually became my traveling companion.

After my dad died, I start asking myself where I would be when I died. In a hospital? At home? My heart would pound wildly as I would think about it. I spent those days feeling raw and ripped open. I finally found my answer to this question—I would be in meditation. I may not have a choice as to the physical location—it may be too low or too high—but I hope I have my block!

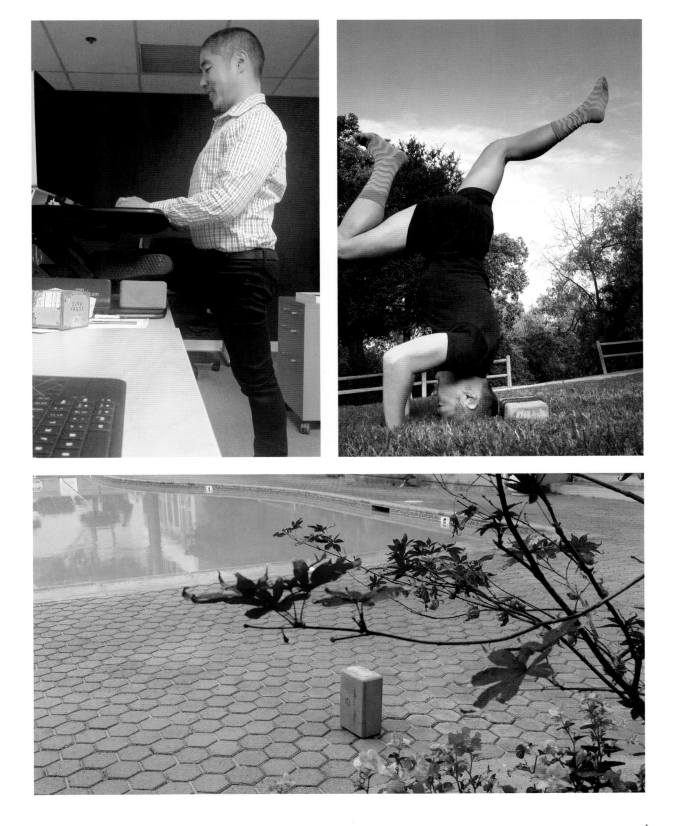

"Practicing long timings in inversions helps me soothe and balance my emotions."

Patricia Walden

CAMBRIDGE, MASSACHUSETTS | YOGA TEACHER

A prominent figure in the evolution of American yoga, Patricia brings a depth of wisdom, keen observation, and elegant refinement to her teaching and her own practice. She holds a senior advanced certificate in the Iyengar method.

My practice has helped me cope with the sadness I have felt since the passing of my beloved Guruji. Since his death, I have been feeling quite introverted and drawn to practicing long timings in inversions, which have always helped me soothe and balance my emotions. Inversions often take me beyond my ordinary mind and bring me into a meditative state. I am able to cut the "threads" to the external world and rest in the present.

Yoga helped me heal from depression in my thirties. I was physically and mentally weak, so learning to do arm balances and backbends was transformative. Practicing them regularly helped me cultivate courage, inner strength, and a healthy sense of self. It was during

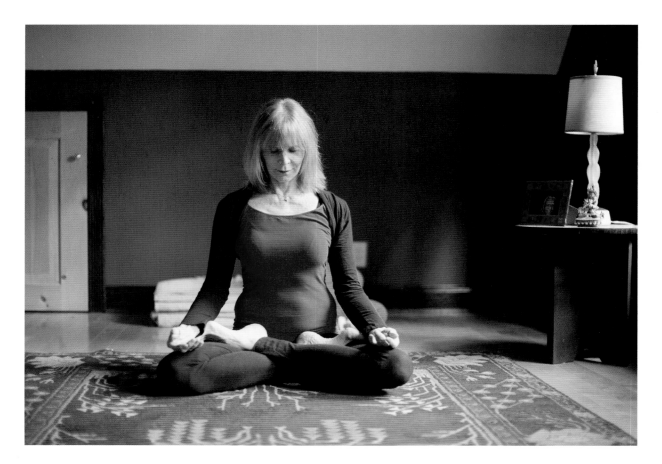

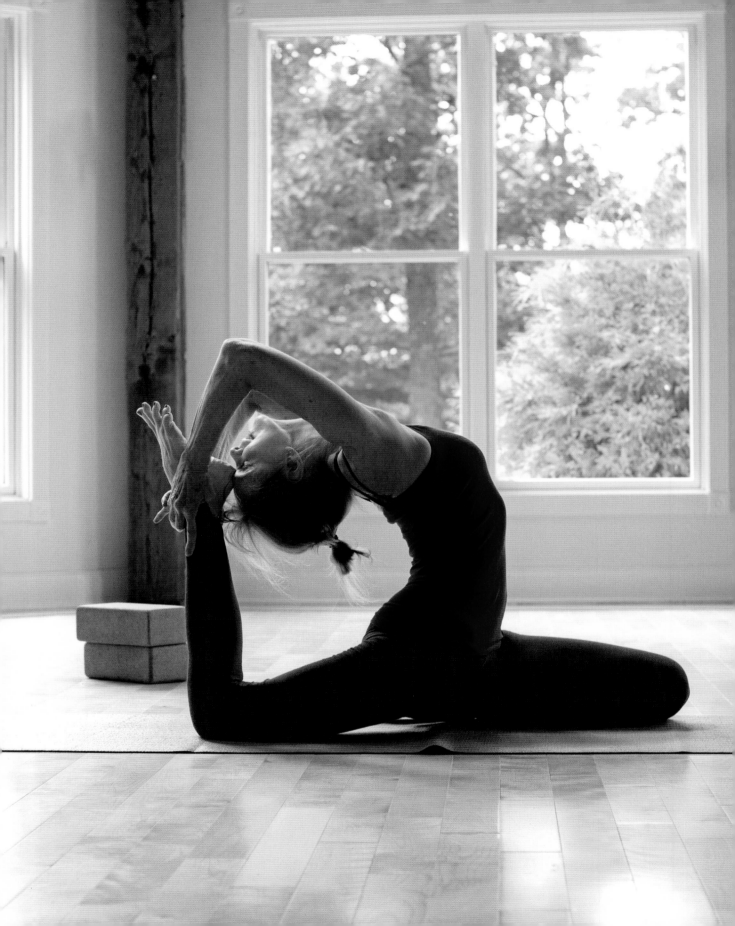

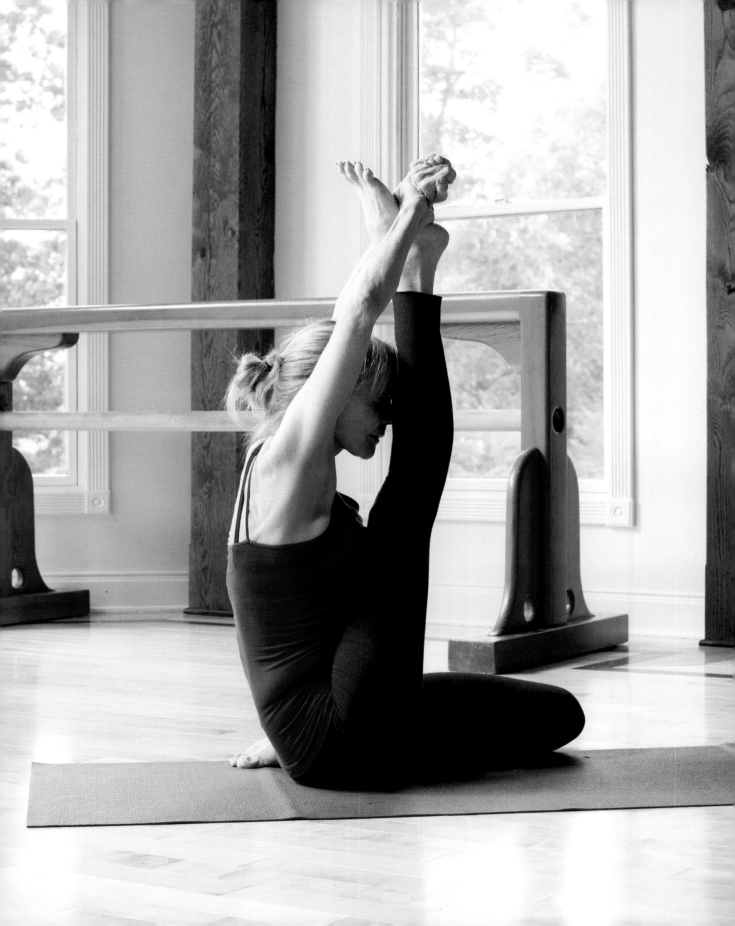

those difficult years that I learned that what you do with your body can have a powerful effect on your mind.

Sometimes I wake up stiff and wonder, what will my body feel like if I start doing backbends? Then I start my practice, and 20 minutes into it I feel younger and forget that I'm almost seventy years old. Inevitably, the power of yoga takes over and I feel ageless!

Not long ago, I went to my mat with the intention of doing a series of dropbacks from Tadasana (Mountain Pose). I thought, gosh, I'm over sixty-five. I don't know if I'm up to it. Then I remembered that Iyengar did 108 dropbacks—on his eightieth birthday! His feet were planted; they didn't move. I realized it was my mind, not my body, saying I couldn't do it. As we get older, we have to be careful of the tricks our minds can play on us. Sometimes your mind tells you to be careful for good reason, but sometimes it's telling you that your body can't do something that it *can* do.

I never let my age define me or hold me back. Many of my asanas continue to improve, which is wonderful, but that's no longer my reason for practicing. At the beginning, I had a very physical practice and my main interest was to improve. This was an important stage to go through. Practicing to improve cultivated willpower and created an inner fire. My poses are better, more integrated, than when I was younger. My flexibility and strength are more balanced, as are my effort and relaxation. I try never to take my body for granted. I feel such gratitude that yoga came into my life and that my body still enjoys bending forward and backward.

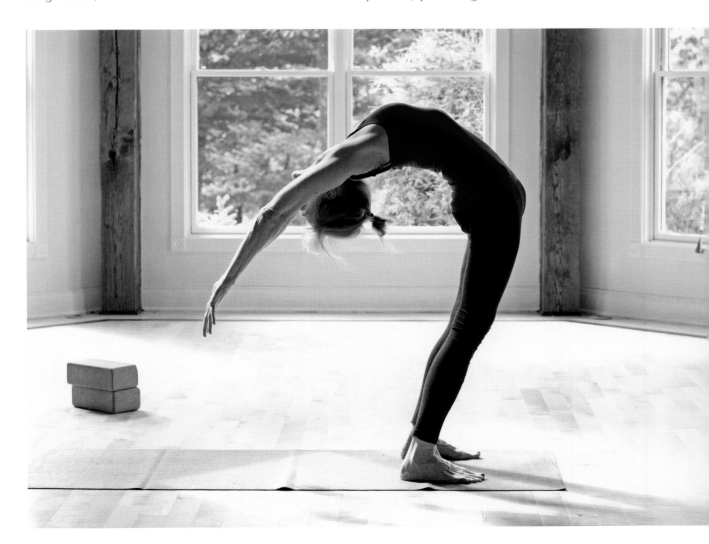

PATRICIA'S SAMPLE PRACTICE

It sometimes takes willpower and self-discipline to show up on our mats no matter what. Willpower isn't just something that exists in the mind; it lives in the body as well. Whenever you go against that inner voice that says, "I can't," or "I'm too tired," you charge the battery of willpower and build a reservoir of resolve to draw upon whenever you need it. Practice these five poses at least three times a week with loving attention and affection for your body.

☙ Virabhadrasana (Warrior Poses)
These poses can help you develop the courage, focus, and determination you need to deal with life's challenges.

☙ Adho Mukha Svanasana
(Downward-Facing Dog)
If your mind is scattered, it's hard to commit to practice. When that happens, do just one pose, like Downward-Facing Dog, a pose that requires muscular effort to hold.

☙ Chaturanga Dandasana
(Four-Limbed Staff Pose)
It's tempting to move quickly through physical or emotional discomfort. But facing difficulty head on cultivates willpower. Commit to doing this pose slowly and deliberately once a day for a week.

☙ Ustrasana (Camel Pose)
Backbends help us face our fears—or the unknown—with a fierce heart. Hold this pose for a few breaths longer than you think you can.

☙ Paschimottanasana
(Seated Forward Bend)
Forward bends cultivate the will to be still. When challenging thoughts or emotions arise, focus on slow, soft, deep exhalations.

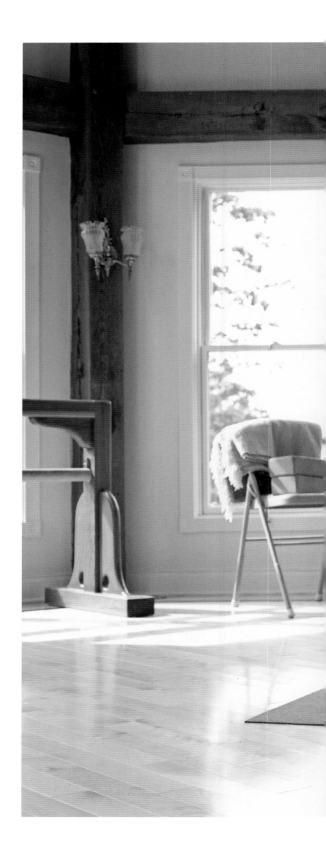

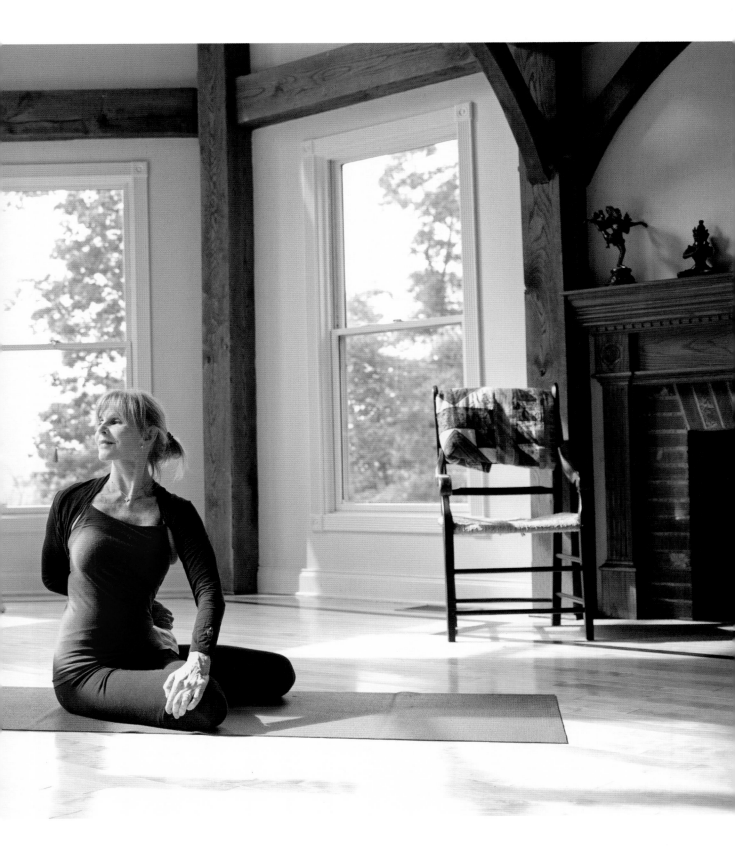

> *"My home practice has cultivated a healthier and more accurate awareness of self."*

James Brown

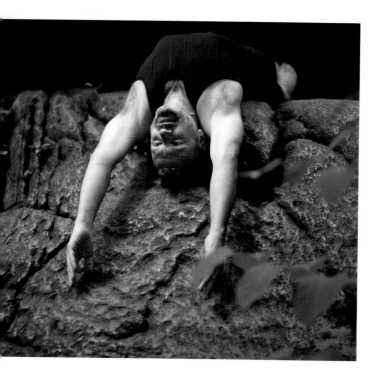

LOS ANGELES, CALIFORNIA | YOGA TEACHER

By teaching precise technique, fluency in biomechanics, and the practical application of the *Yoga Sutra*, James presents asana as a way to make a happier life. His influences include his longtime teacher, YogaWorks founder Maty Ezraty.

At the moment, I live in a house in Los Angeles that has a dedicated yoga room. There is nothing in it except what I need to practice, which is helpful because it allows for boundaries in space within which I only do yoga. But it isn't really the room or its contents that make the space special; it's the practice that happens there. The space, ideally, provides a container for practice that doesn't get in the way of the practice itself.

I travel a lot and don't always have access to my dedicated home practice space. In those cases, the ideal is to have any practice-sized space that can be carved out and used only for practice. It doesn't even need to have walls or a door. When I have this option, I keep my yoga mat unrolled there so it's clear what the space is for (and to remind me to practice).

If I could choose any kind of space for practice, it would be outdoors in a quiet, private place on a hot, humid morning. So, on one of my many trips to New York City, I was delighted to discover the Ramble, a section in Central Park that was designed to appear as a wild and uncultivated forest. Although very busy pathways are less than a minute away, this area, populated by huge boulders, is most often nearly silent and practically deserted. The boulders became the platform—and the props I needed—for my practice. I came to it whenever I could.

My yoga practice, as defined by the *Yoga Sutra*, is an attempt to steady the mind. A few years ago, I discovered that a particularly stagnant period in my practice had been initiated by a gradual blurring of

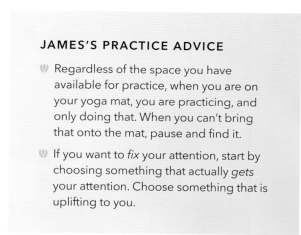

JAMES'S PRACTICE ADVICE

- Regardless of the space you have available for practice, when you are on your yoga mat, you are practicing, and only doing that. When you can't bring that onto the mat, pause and find it.

- If you want to *fix* your attention, start by choosing something that actually *gets* your attention. Choose something that is uplifting to you.

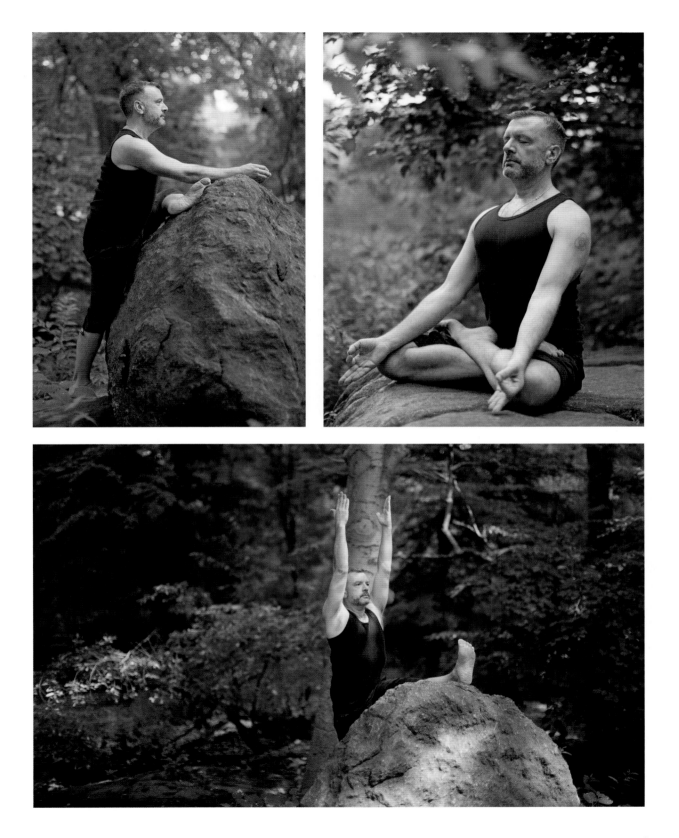

the boundaries between what constitutes designated practice and what does not. My solution was to occupy my mat only when I was there to practice earnestly and skillfully. My self-inflicted rule was that, if I caught myself putting my efforts toward nonpractice distractions, I was to step off my mat and get myself together. I only had to give myself a few of these time-outs before I started opting for earnest practice more consistently.

While there are myriad ways I could practice, I choose to practice asana ninety-nine percent of the time because it is the thing I know the best. The familiarity I find in asana allows me to see how I am different that day, and that informs my efforts. Something less familiar, like chanting or silent meditation, can be a nice shift and bring great calm. But I am less able to steer the practice when I am outside my asana-practitioner skill set. So I pretty much stick to asana, even if that means doing nothing more than a highly focused Corpse Pose.

Shifting my habit to self-practice, done alone without external distraction, was like cleaning a pair of glasses that I didn't realize was dirty. Without the distraction of my ego dealing with the ever-shifting landscape of a group practice, I suddenly saw myself with new clarity. Once that happened, I was hooked for life. My home practice has cultivated a healthier and more accurate awareness of self than the one that I saw when practicing in public.

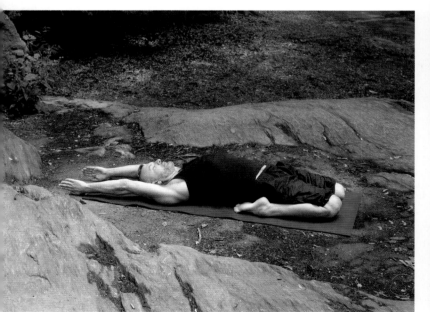

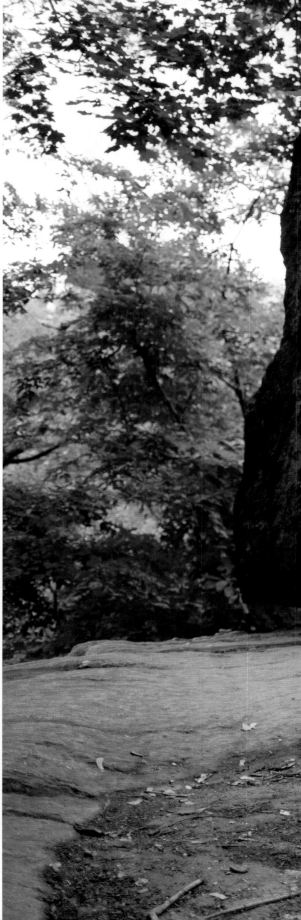

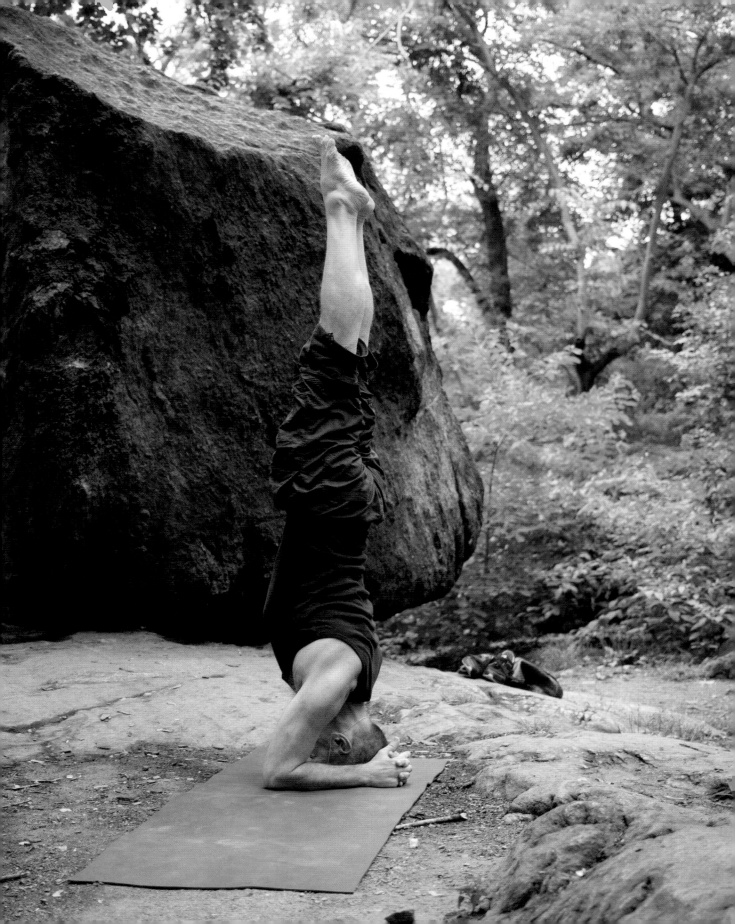

"Right side up, my world is very full. Upside down, it quiets down and empties out."

Justine Wiltshire Cohen

CAMBRIDGE, MASSACHUSETTS | YOGA TEACHER/YOGA STUDIO OWNER

In Justine's crazy, busy life as the owner of Down Under Yoga, teacher, and mother to three young kids, yoga is hardly an indulgence; it's a necessity. Her practice combines a powerful blend of vigorous vinyasa flow and anatomical precision.

Our house is like Grand Central Station. At any given hour of the day, our kitchen witnesses life at its fullest. My two-year-old son pulls his train across the floor, my six-year-old daughter practices piano (adding wildly romantic lyrics to her otherwise classical pieces), and my eight-year-old discusses the battle of Troy over breakfast. My mother-in-law does her weekly inspection of my pantry, tut-tutting that we "waste" money on organics, while discussing World War II with my mother, who grew up in a concentration camp in Shanghai. My father, who is permanently outraged at our crumbling Victorian, fixes up our

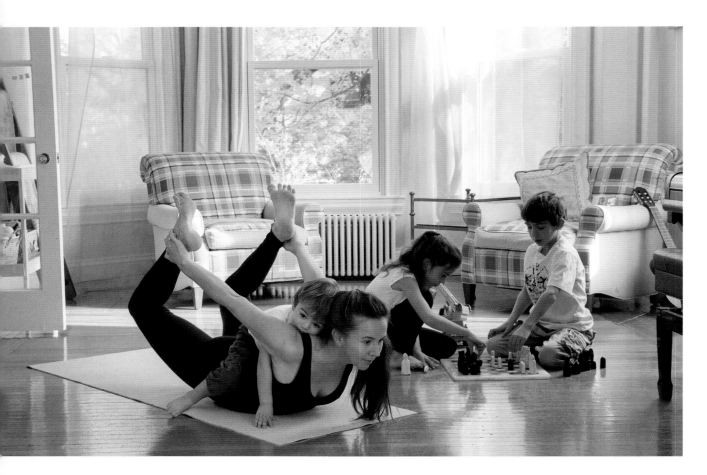

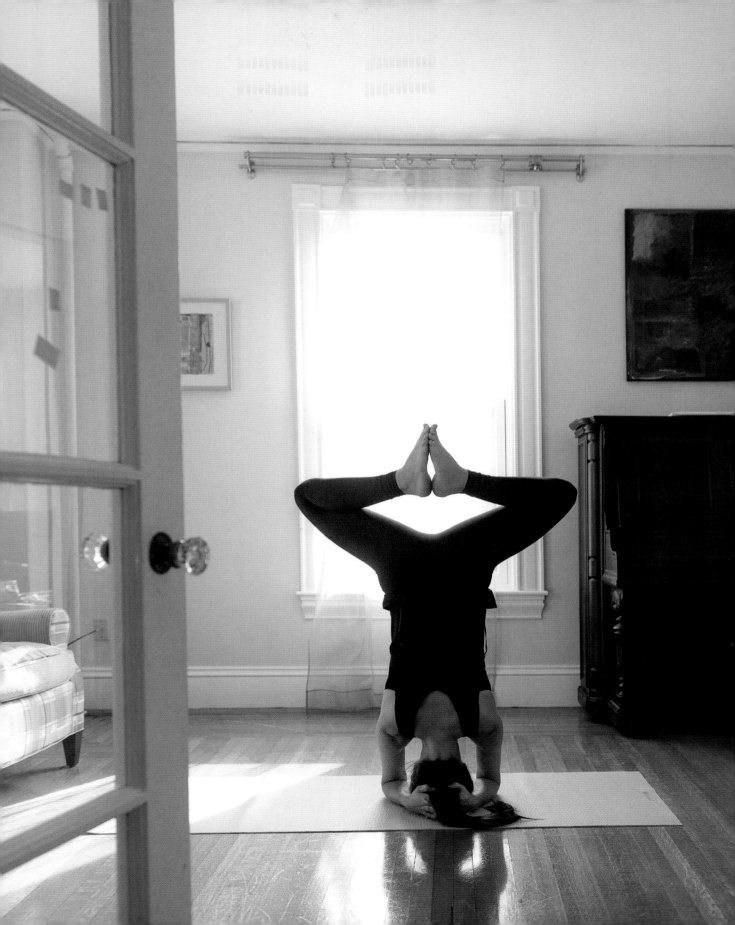

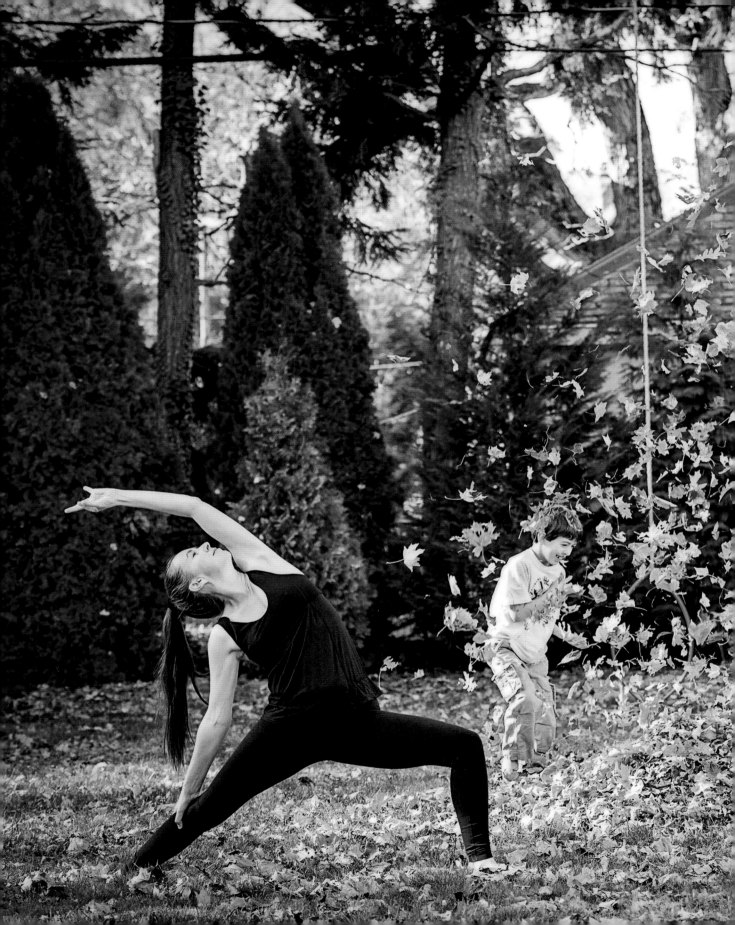

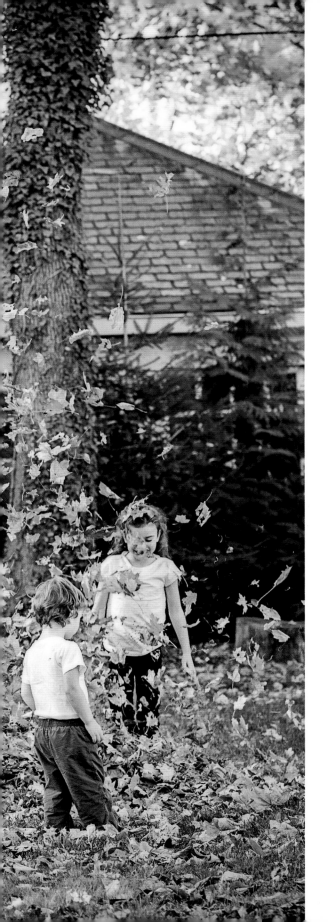

broken back steps, while the eight managers of Down Under Yoga arrive to use our top floor as a "home office." Sometimes if a manager needs a place to live, they move in for a bit—the last manager stayed a year.

Consequently, I love my yoga practice. It is vinyasa based with long inversions. Right side up, my world is very full. Upside down, everything quiets down and empties out. The children on the piano or yelling in the hallway fades into a single pointed focus. I usually have to overcome some initial pang of guilt, the passing thought that yoga is an indulgence or that I should be attending to someone. Then I remember that yoga is not an indulgence; it is a necessity.

Sacred space (like the practice of yoga itself) is created by the quality of your attention, the texture of your breath. The simpler the space, the better—otherwise it takes on a rarified quality or requires certain conditions or accoutrements, all the stuff that practice moves us away from. I love that in the seminal texts the highest form of yoga is not the monk who isolates himself in the cave, free from distraction. The greatest acclaim goes to the practitioner who lives and works in the messiness and complexity of the real world, practicing mindfulness in the midst of love, disappointment, chaos, and convolution.

The beautiful thing about yoga is that it is not an intellectual exercise—it is a sensation-based practice. Asana awakens the physical body and makes it intelligent. But the movement itself is a preparation for stillness. The body never really speaks until it's convinced that you're willing to be quiet enough to listen. Yoga is itself a profound challenge to a culture that values multitasking, sensory overload, and an addictive devotion to technology antithetical to the concept of being present and aware. The children of this generation will need to unlearn much of what they know by the age of eight. They will need to practice how to unplug, to single-task, and to withdraw from endless opportunities for narcissism, distraction, and nonbeing. In such a society, stillness and silence become a radical act of courage, even defiance.

"I might not be in a mood to practice, but once I stand on the mat, I do it."

Kevin Ogutu

NAIROBI, KENYA | YOGA TEACHER

An Africa Yoga Project teacher, Kevin begins his day by doing his own home practice—sometimes indoors and sometimes on the rooftop. That time on his own mat helps him connect joyously and calmly with his students.

I am the most free and relaxed when I practice at home. Sometimes in my home practice, I work on awakening the spine. I also like to work on grounding because I must meet and face different kinds of people in the course of the day.

My yoga mat makes me practice; I don't roll it or pack it. I leave it spread out. I get out of bed and step right onto the mat. I might not be in a mood to practice, but once I stand on the mat, I do it.

I have classes that I lead every day and when I lead those classes I connect with my practice in the morning. I figure out what needs to be worked on, and it relates to my morning practice. I face my students with calmness because I did my practice.

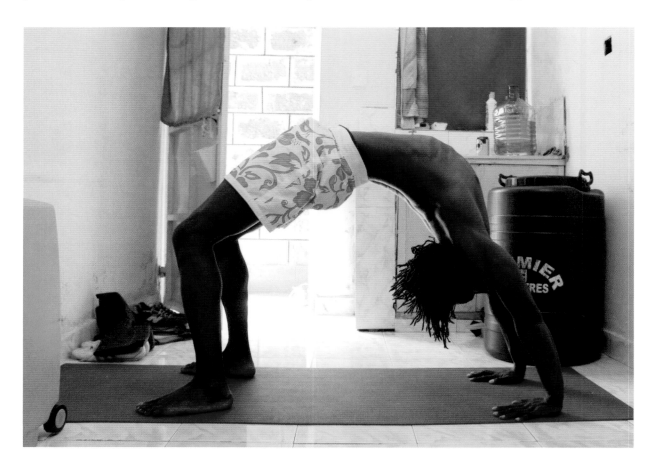

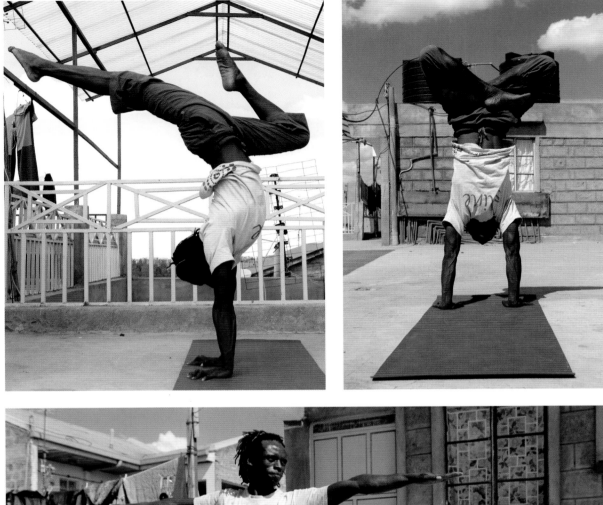

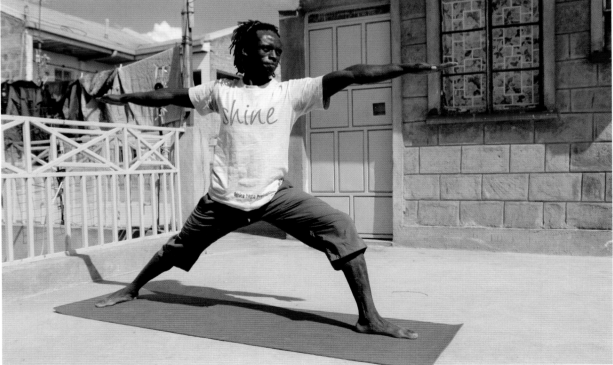

*"The great thing about not knowing what to do
is that you actually don't know what to do!"*

Rodney Yee & Colleen Saidman-Yee

NEW YORK & EAST HAMPTON, NEW YORK | YOGA TEACHERS/YOGA STUDIO CO-OWNERS

One of the most well-known yoga couples in America, Rodney and Colleen teach yoga to bring philosophy into action and unveil the natural beauty of our spirits. They codirect the health and wellness initiative of Urban Zen Foundation.

It's hard to talk about practice if you don't first talk about what you're trying to do. Of course, we both like pushing and pulling, trying to find out where the tension is in the body; we still like stretching and flexibility, range of motion, and strength. But as the practice goes on, there's something else that you're searching for. There's some sublime taste; you know, like a really fine wine. There are certain things that a home practice exposes that might not surface otherwise. That's really the core of practice: who are you and what needs to be expressed? Yoga is the tool, not the end in itself; it's a craft in which to express something, communicate it freely, and then through that expression have connection with others.

RODNEY: Why home practice? It's *only* home practice. When you go to class you get ideas, you hear another voice, you break open another way of seeing something. But without home practice, there's really no way to digest that. Without making it your own,

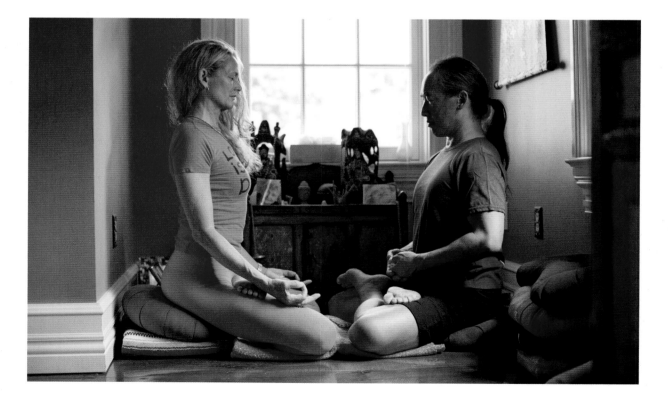

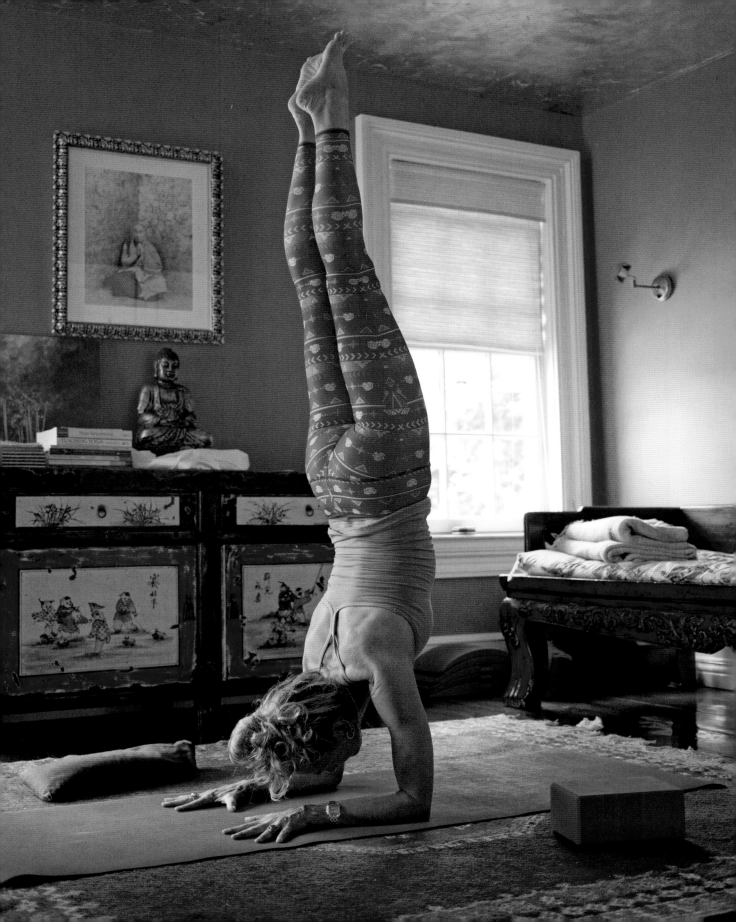

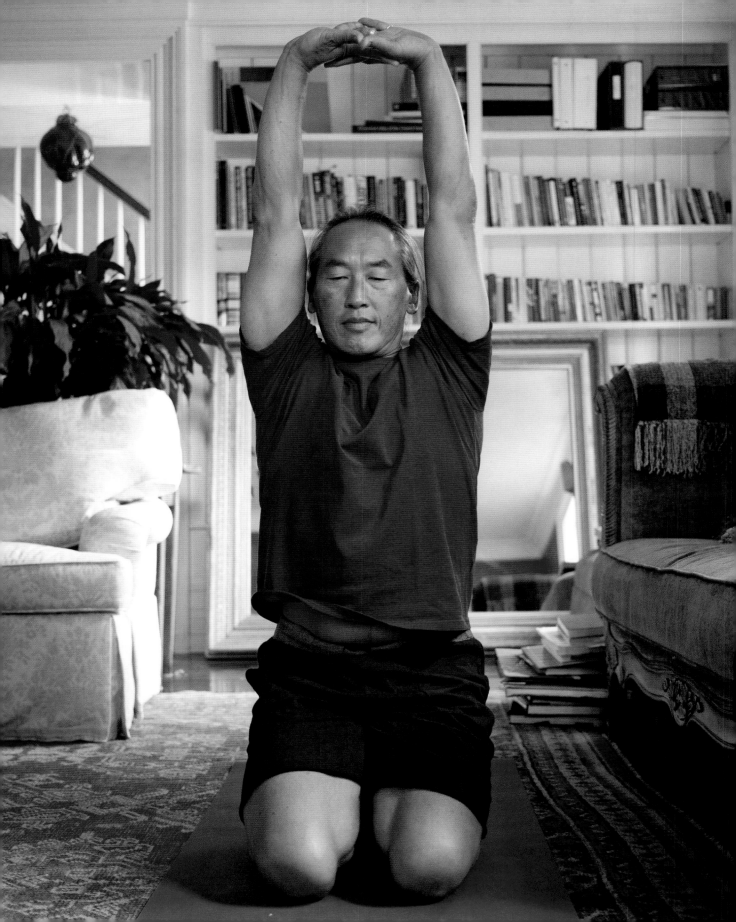

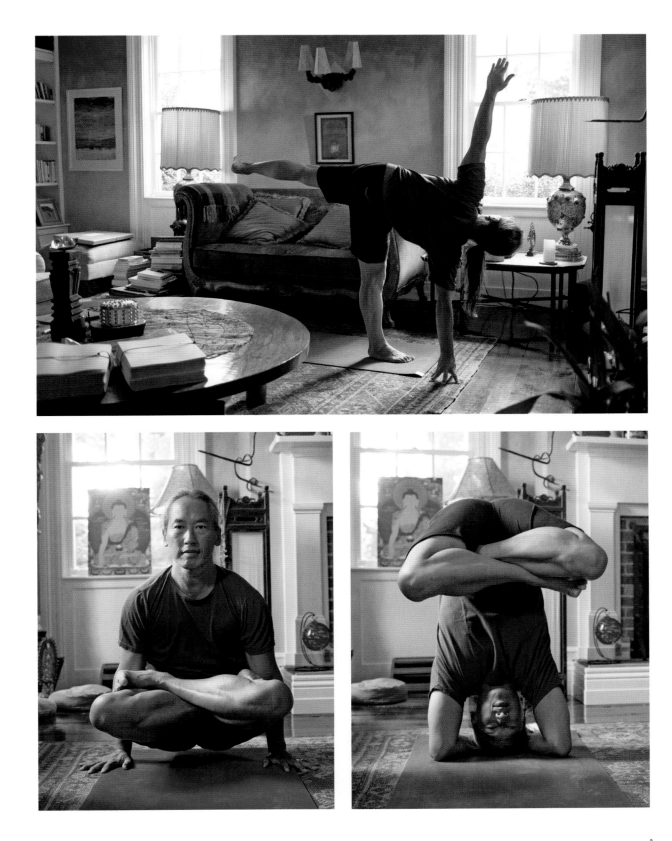

yoga doesn't mean anything. It becomes just an exercise class. There's a certain aloneness and creativity that comes out of home practice. To evoke it in your own space and time and listen to yourself—there's an essence there that can't be cracked open in a class.

Home practice is frustrating a lot of times because it's not someone telling you what to do and you following. It's picking the skin off your feet, picking your nose, and then doing a pose. You don't do that in someone else's class, but you do in home practice. I remember watching Prashant (B. K. S. Iyengar's grandson) practicing in India. He would hang upside down for a while, then look out the window, do another pose,

and then walk around. His practice seemed like a way for him to align with the world. For me, it's like having yoga consciousness throughout the day. Whether or not I succeed and can be calm and centered is not the point. The point is being thrown off and noticing it.

Home practice gives us that extra moment of authentic practice. We have the opportunity to respond with our true nature in this present moment—not how it's been identified before; not how we were before; not how we hope to be; not how we intend to be. Our authentic self, in the present moment.

COLLEEN: In home practice, you get to discover what *you* need for balance rather than let someone else decide what's going to bring you balance. So if you haven't slept and you want to lie down and do Savasana with tons of weights on . . . that's yoga! But if you don't ever do that, how are you going to even understand who you are or how you've evolved?

Rodney and I do pranayama to discover where we are at a particular moment. Looking at your breath can help you very much. You know when you're forcing, when you're holding, when you're not being honest.

Home practice allows you to be who you want to be. You can do what you want to do. You can become who you want to become. Doing your own practice helps you unwind tension so that there's space. We talk about this all the time. You can create that internal, nonjudgmental space so that there's room for your bad hip, your good shoulder, your rage, and your joy.

RODNEY: The great thing about not knowing what to do is that you actually don't know what to do! And the problem is not that we as teachers can't give beginners a sequence to do so they can get on with it—we can. The problem is that they think they should *do* something, anything, other than not knowing.

As a teacher, you sometimes want your students to be frustrated on some level, to be "not knowing" and just sitting there picking their toes. And then other times, you want them to do a certain set of poses. So on days one, two, and three, do this. And then on day four, be frustrated, be curious, and create your own sequence.

COLLEEN: On a practical level, I would encourage very beginning students to start with standing poses,

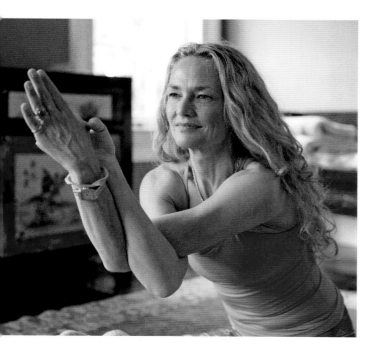

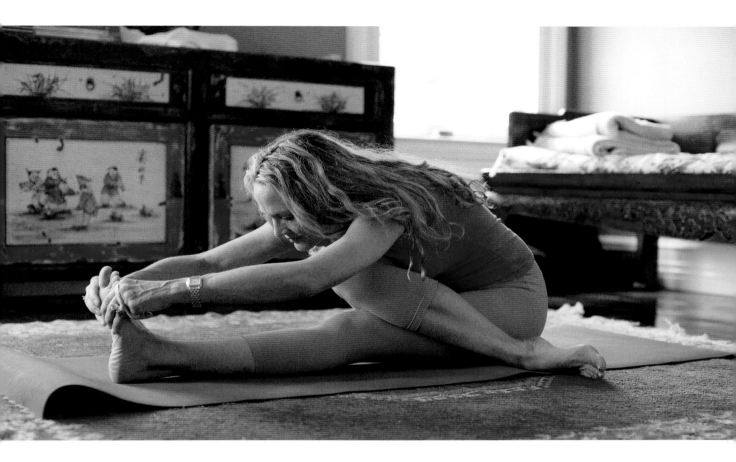

ones they can do themselves, because it's a lot easier to avoid getting hurt. Sometimes very advanced practitioners are not that interested in doing anything at home because there's no audience. I would actually give advanced students a set sequence to do with standing poses, open twists, and backbends. And it would end with pranayama, at least a 5-minute sit, and a 15-minute Savasana.

RODNEY: Advanced practice is subtle; it's in the minutia of something. It's not something that's loud. It's not complicated contortions. It's a nuance of resistance within the prana that's being observed. For advanced practitioners, I would say it's good that your work ethic is strong, but it's also important to find your passion. Sometimes you have to sit still long enough for something genuine to arise and then have the courage to follow that arising voice. And it's not the same every day. It's a listening game. After the listening, true activity actually unfolds in a natural and harmonious way.

For me, something specific often arises. I'll sit and then make a cup of coffee. I'll read the news in a squat or Child's Pose. And, all of a sudden, a message will appear, like a spontaneous fortune cookie, and say, you should practice twists today!

COLLEEN'S PRACTICE ADVICE

- ◊ Be consistent, but don't be overly ambitious. Start with 20 minutes a day, even if you spend the entire 20 minutes lying on your back.

- ◊ Spend time *after* you practice observing the effects of what you've just done. For example, if you do a closed twist and forward bend sequence, how do you feel energetically and physically afterward?

"Yoga helped me get through a prison sentence and helps me deal with life's daily struggles."

Talon Demeo

SAN FRANCISCO, CALIFORNIA | TATTOO ARTIST/MUSICIAN

Tattoo artist and punk-rock musician Talon has everything he needs in his studio—his work, his home, and his yoga mat—to keep him feeling more grounded and healthier, and to help him stay in the moment.

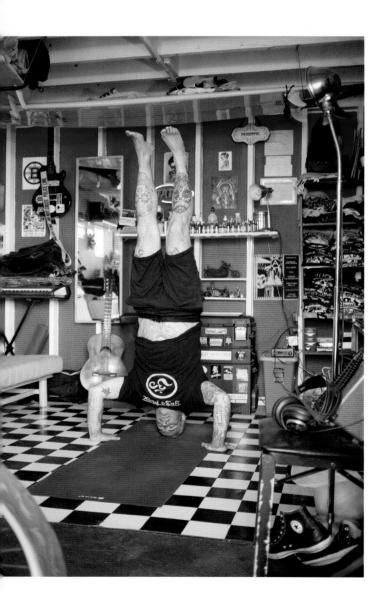

I found yoga while I was in prison in California. Someone gave me a book called *We're All Doing Time: A Guide to Getting Free* by Bo Lozoff and it had a chapter on yoga with about ten poses. When I paroled, I met Khristine Jones (of Yoga Punx) and she taught me everything else I know. Her class is my favorite. She plays punk rock and we do an hour vinyasa flow.

I practice at my tattoo studio, New Approach Ink, every morning. I live there, too, so I do a morning practice. Yoga helped me get through a three-year prison sentence. And yoga continues to help me deal with life's daily struggles. I suffer from lower back pain because I herniated a disk in 2004. So I do my yoga routine every morning just so I can relieve the chronic pain that I live with every day, instead of taking pain medication.

It's hard to stay consistent. For some reason, I'll go days or even a week without practicing, which is crazy because I always feel better after yoga. You'd think I'd always be willing to feel better! I want to be more spiritually fit. I'm on a personal journey to become healthier—mind, body, and soul.

TALON'S PRACTICE ADVICE

- Do yoga at your own pace. It's your practice . . . not a competition.
- You can push yourself, but ultimately it's just about being in the moment.

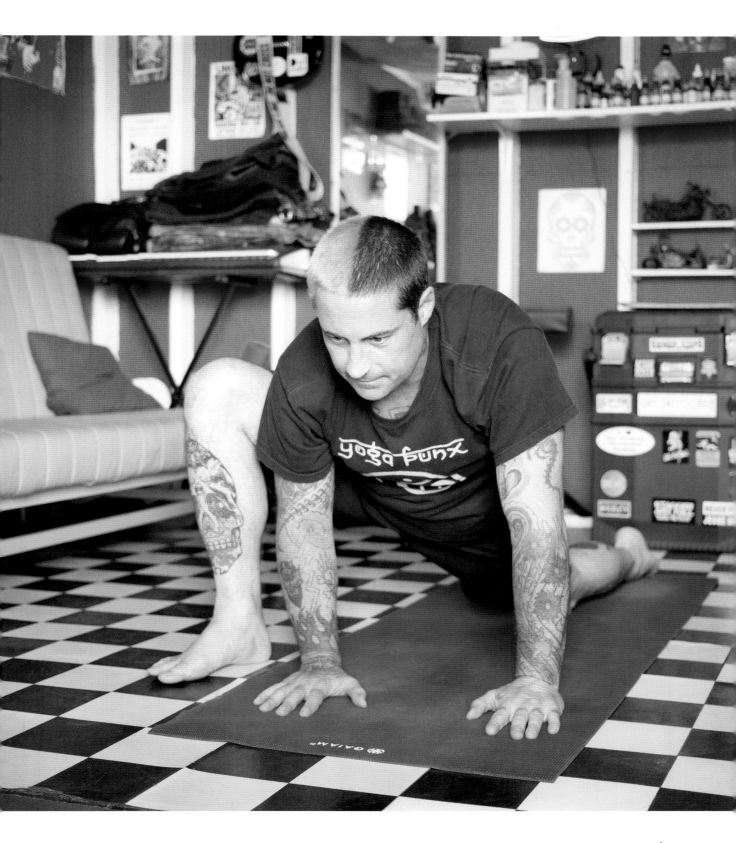

> *"Anything you do in daily life can be sacred, and that makes your home practice unique."*

Maya Kanako

OSAKA, JAPAN | YOGA TEACHER

An OM yoga teacher in Osaka, Japan, Maya shares her daily practice with her cats and employs everything from doorknobs to counters and window ledges to create a home practice that supports her life.

Not everyone in Japan can afford a two-bedroom apartment, not to mention having an extra room just for yoga. If you want to practice yoga at home, you may need to remove some clutter first so you have enough floor space and you won't bump into anything during your practice.

I use whatever things I find in my small apartment that I think will work for my practice. For example, I

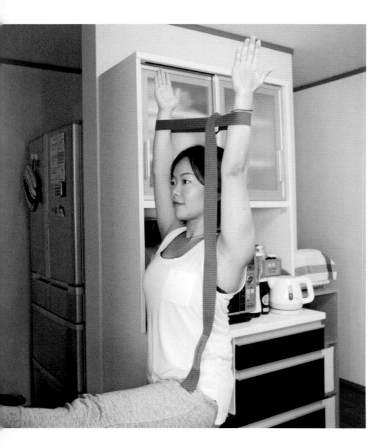

use a doorknob and a yoga belt for a makeshift rope wall to support my Downward-Facing Dog. And I use a window ledge or the edge of my kitchen sink to stretch and strengthen my legs to prepare for standing poses.

You don't need to have a special yoga space to make your home practice special. I would rather focus on how to use the space I do have and how to make my practice more "down to earth."

I usually start my day on the mat. My cats wake me up every morning, no matter what. It may sound cute, but it's usually just a "Is food ready yet?" plea. After I get up, I feed them, play with them, and lounge around with them on a *tatami* (straw-mat) floor. Then, I start my daily practice. I clean the room, roll out my mat, and just see what happens. It's as simple as brushing my teeth. Anything you do in your daily life can be sacred, and that makes your home practice unique and creative. Yoga means everything and you can find yoga in everything!

MAYA'S PRACTICE ADVICE

- Make sure your home practice supports your life. Try not to feel pressured or let yoga take over your life, and don't do anything that doesn't feel right.

- If you are completely new to yoga, take some beginner classes taught by a teacher you like before you start practicing at home. Otherwise, you'll never know if you are doing something wrong or harmful.

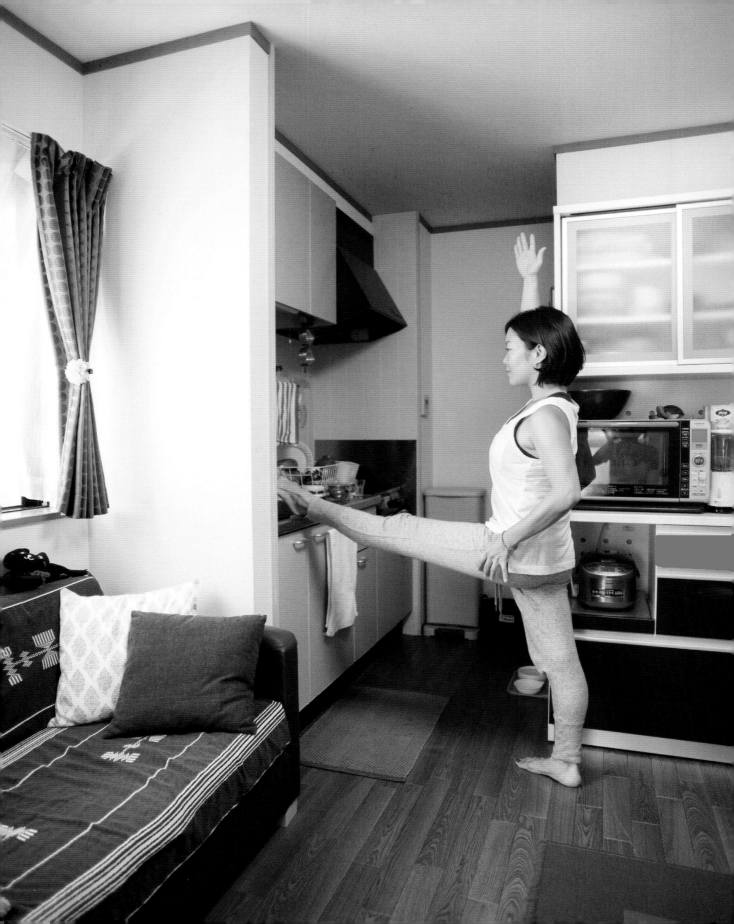

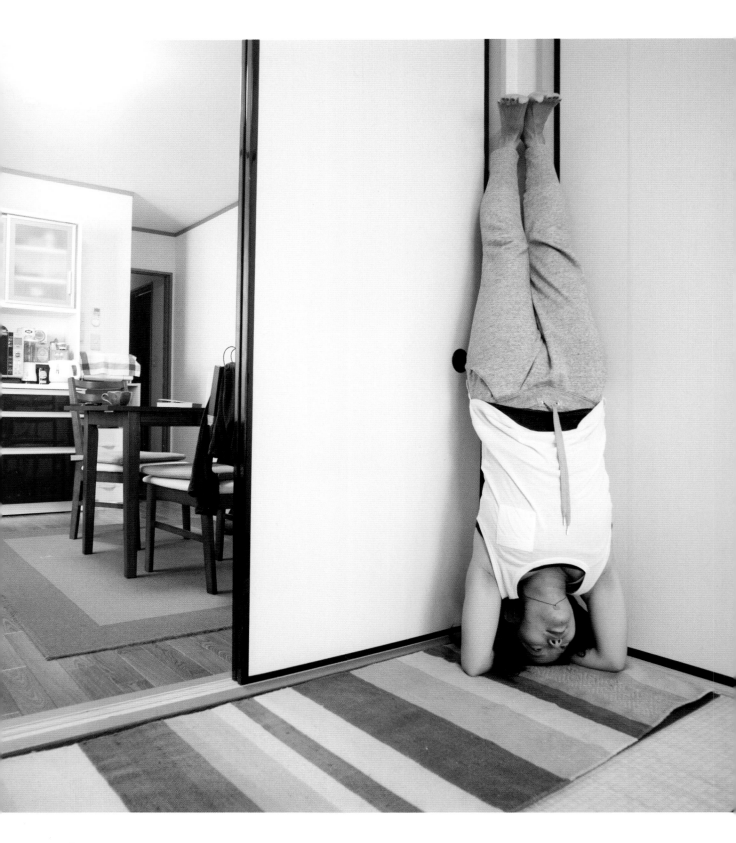

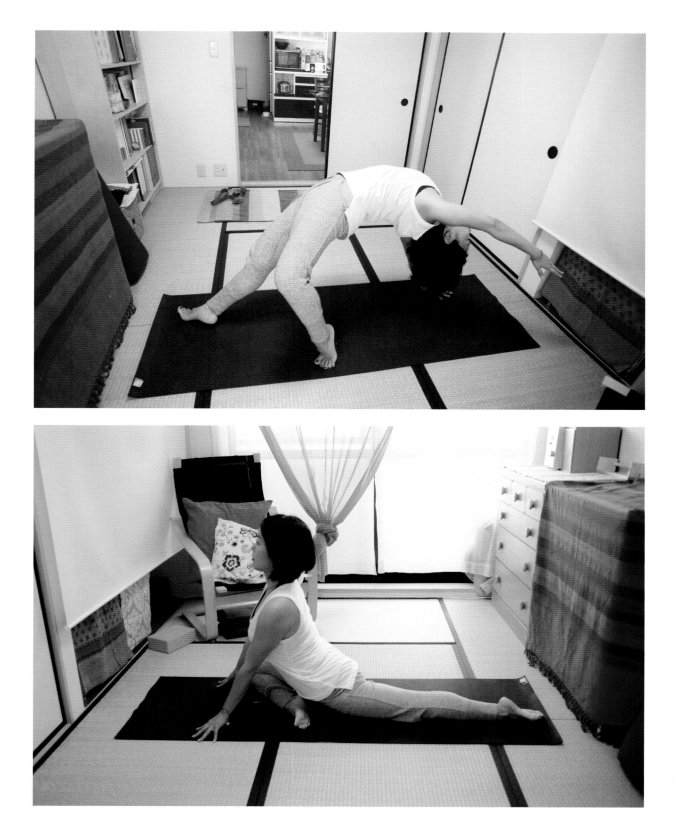

> *"Ultimately, my teaching is a reflection of what my practice provides me in daily life."*

Jason Crandell

SAN FRANCISCO, CALIFORNIA | YOGA TEACHER

Jason's classes integrate power yoga, anatomical precision, and mindfulness teachings to create an efficient, balanced practice. He offers tools to help you stress less, communicate more effectively, and embrace and enjoy who you are.

We own a small home in San Francisco, which means all rooms are multipurpose rooms—especially with a toddler. That also means I don't have a room just for my practice. Come to think of it, in seventeen years of practicing yoga at home, I've never had a separate space. Currently, I practice in three separate rooms depending on my mood: in our front room/office if I need a little more space or quiet time or if I want greater intensity in my practice; in our bedroom if I want to check in with my online community, since it's private and the Wi-Fi is strong; and in our living room if I want to practice and interact with my family at the same time. It's our daughter's favorite room to practice in, so this usually means forward bends and hip openers while playing with Legos or doing crafts. I love it because it feels like honest, comfortable time with my family.

My practice has helped me navigate difficult periods for as long as I've had a practice. It provides me with an opportunity to feel whatever is present without judging it. It also provides me with the tools to manage my nervous system and helps me minimize my

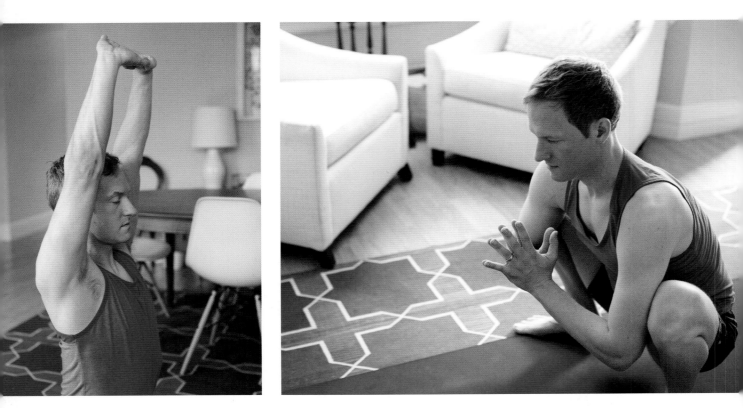

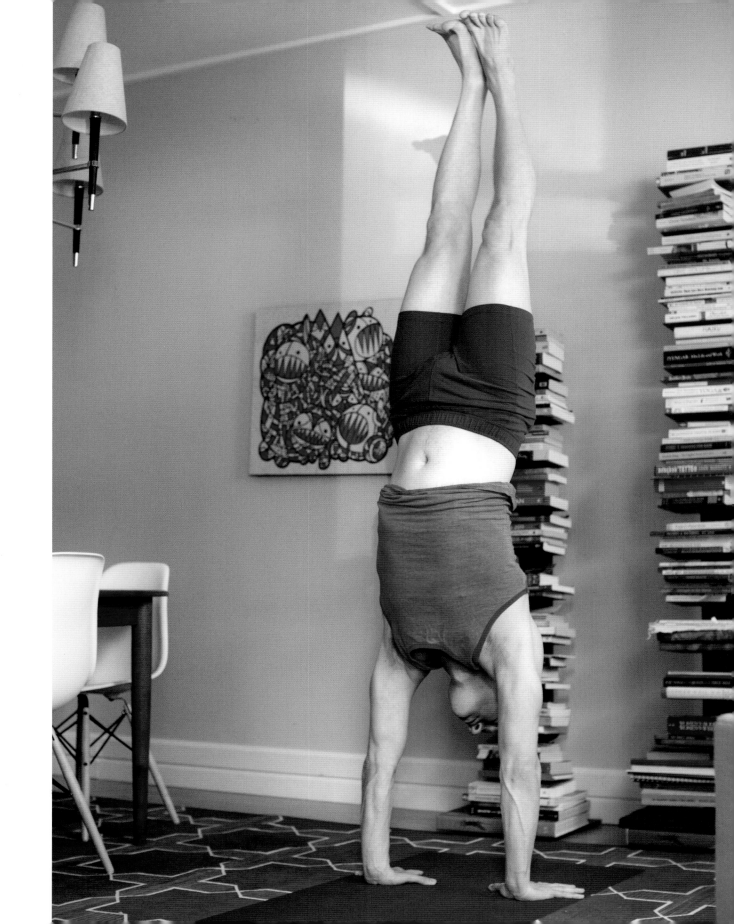

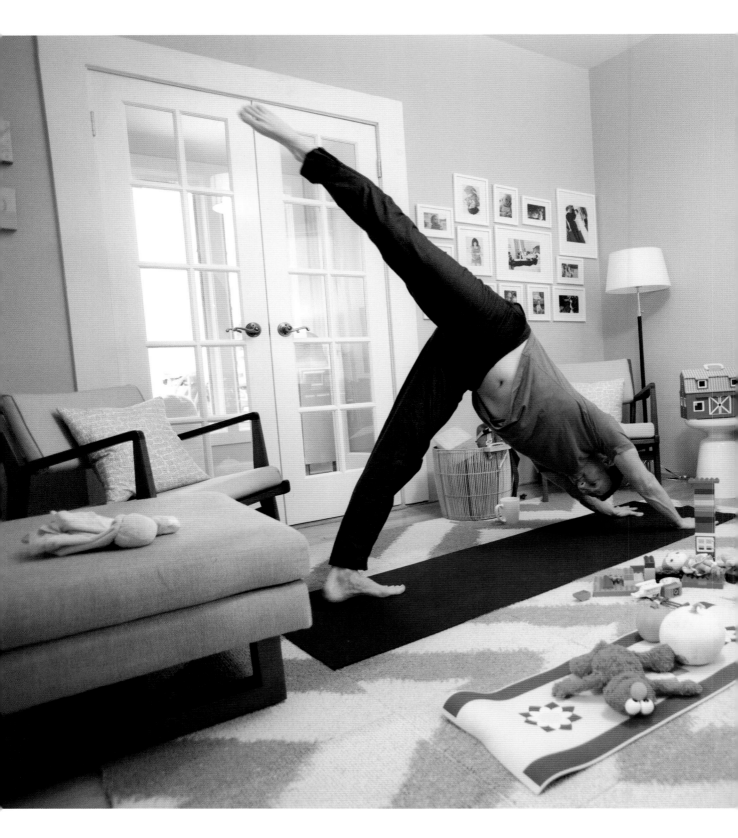

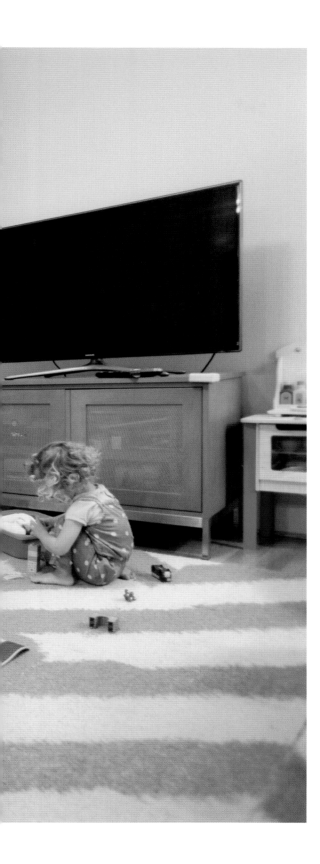

reaction to events. It has made me more steady, calm, and focused in the presence of challenging phases.

I'm always happy to practice and rarely go through periods these days where I don't feel like practicing. Sure, sometimes I want an easy, quiet, effortless practice. If this is the case, I simply give in and lie over a couple of bolsters in a restorative practice or set my timer and do a yin practice. Other days, if I feel like working harder, I'll crank out a vinyasa practice. Since I have a big range in my practice with regards to intensity, it's easy to savor most any day on the mat.

Yoga continues to keep me relatively grounded, content, and sane. It helps regulate my mood, energy, and focus. It allows me to teach with a high degree of integrity and authenticity because, ultimately, my teaching is a reflection of what my practice provides me in daily life.

Jamie Lamke

SAUSALITO, CALIFORNIA | YOGA TEACHER

Carpenter, dancer, and dedicated yogi, Jamie's strengths are his grasp of the fundamentals, compassion for pain, and understanding of human challenges. A student of Manouso Manos, Jamie teaches Iyengar yoga in the Bay Area.

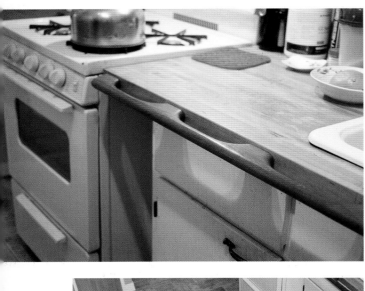

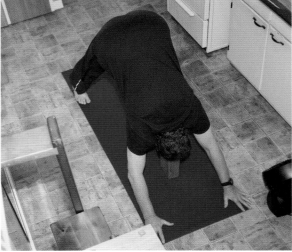

Since I live in a tiny studio, with not much room to practice, I needed to carve out some space for yoga. I chose my kitchen. When I first moved in, the all-white skinny kitchen was fully carpeted and tricked out with 1950s-style, avocado-colored, full-sized appliances. So the first thing I did was pull out the big ugly refrigerator and convert that space into a combination pantry and yoga prop closet. I replaced the fridge with an under-the-counter variety, traded in the big stove for a smaller one, and swapped the old Formica countertops with butcher block. Then I made a teak grab rail that I bolted to the front edge of the counter, which I use as a barre.

Once I had all that done, I installed Iyengar-style baseboards and asphalt linoleum, which turns out to be the best floor I've ever practiced on. It has perfect traction for bare feet, and it matches your body temperature in Savasana within seconds. No more cold floor.

I got rid of the old harsh, glaring globe light and put in modern track lights on a dimmer switch. I painted the whole room a cheery lemon yellow with white trim, installed a ropes wall for Yoga Karunta, and put up a full set of anatomy charts for reference. Then I was all set to practice and to compose classes.

Full disclosure: I'm no construction rookie. In my carpenter days, I helped design and build a half dozen yoga, dance, and martial arts studios, and consulted on several more. But this is the only thing I've ever designed and built exclusively for myself, using the existing space to the best of my ability, and I must admit that I still walk in the door sometimes, look at what I've created, and think, "Cool!"

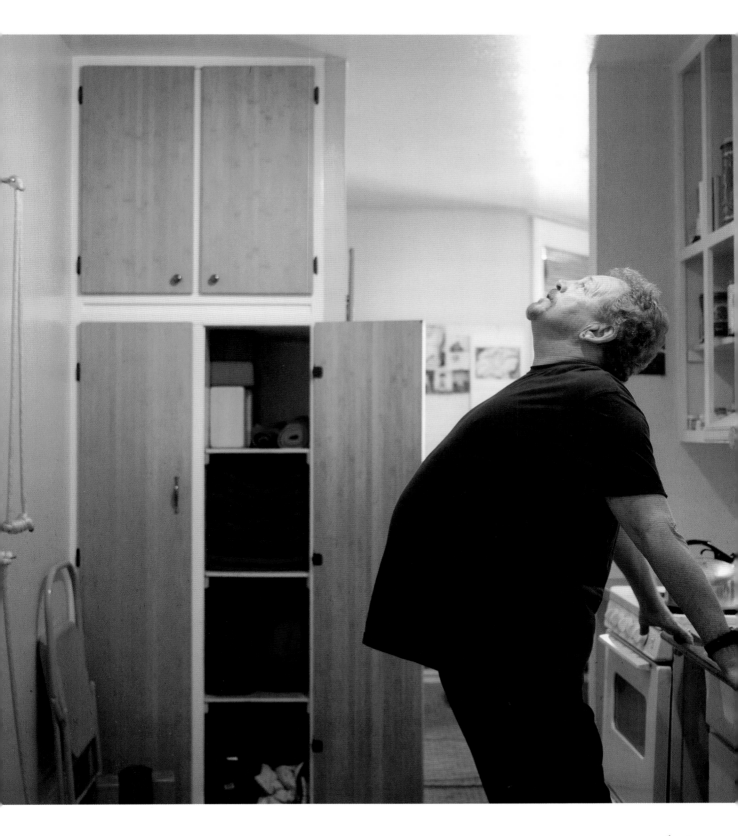

> *"Yoga is your time to see who you are and how you are and examine your fears."*

Annie Carpenter

OAKLAND, CALIFORNIA | YOGA TEACHER

Annie's SmartFlow style reflects both her love of movement and rigorous discipline, along with a passion for creativity and metaphor. Her influences include Integral and Iyengar yoga, and Maty Ezraty and Chuck Miller, founders of YogaWorks.

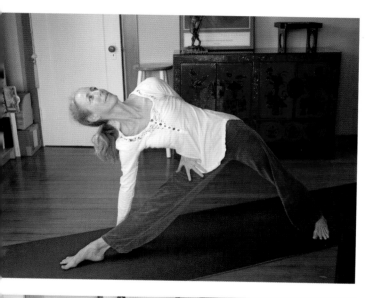

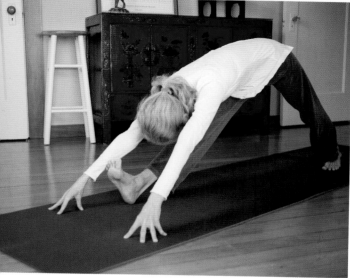

I practice for self-inquiry. As time goes on, the process of inquiry has become such a driving factor in everything I do. How is this action serving me or how is it in my way? How am I experiencing this in the moment? Is it helpful or not? If not, what do I need to do to make it helpful? Or, perhaps, is it possible for me to be OK with it and not necessarily need to change it?

All that has taken time. Some things I live with easily even if they're not the most comfortable things. Some things are ready to be shifted and changed and that feels good and positive and uplifting. Some things aren't. That inquiry of acceptance and the capacity to be OK with things as they are is what informs what my practice looks like every day.

Of course, I have great fun when I get into an inquiry that actually leads down a path, especially if it's a newer path—oh, look at this! Then I usually stay with it for a few days. It may shift a little, but it goes deeper. And sometimes it leads me down a completely different path. It's fun!

In my thirties and even into my forties, I needed to do every big pose I could, every single day of my life. Moving in every direction, every day, looking for that extreme edge. After a while, that's just not as comfortable, nor is it as interesting, as looking at what I call "the ten percent before the end." When we're younger, going all the way to that extreme edge—the one hundred percent—is exhilarating. But now I put my effort into a particular part of my body, then I sort of pull back five or ten percent. I'm fascinated by that in-between place. That process is way more interesting, and, frankly, much deeper, than extreme edges.

In the morning, I'll sit first to see how I'm doing and what I need. I'll choose a pranayama to balance

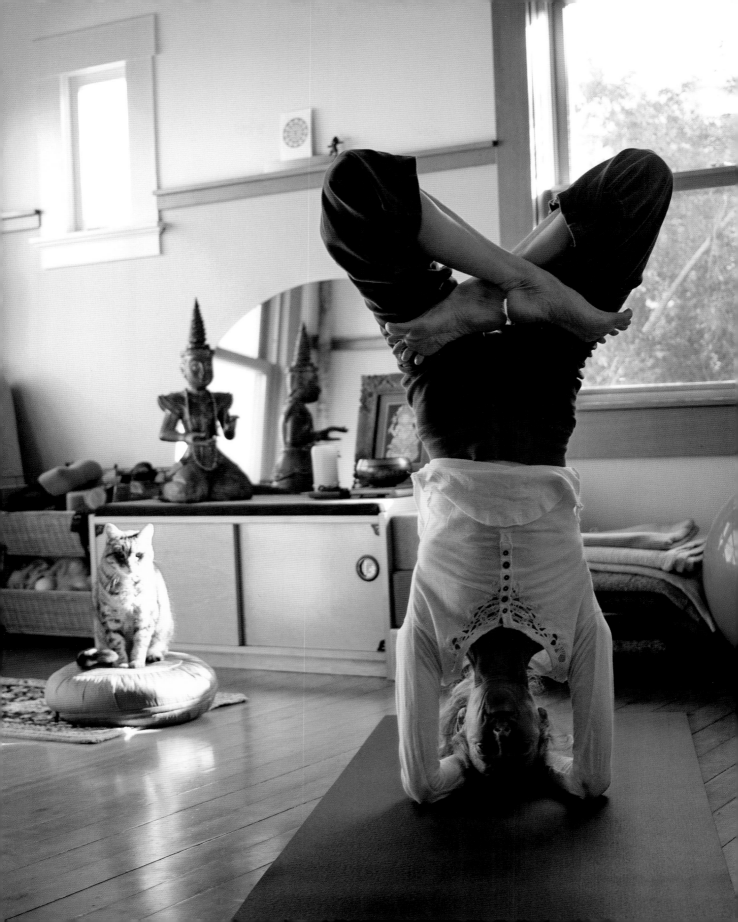

my energy, depending on whether it's scattered or more focused, and I'll do it for 5 minutes, maybe 10 minutes, so that when I sit in meditation, my mind can be a little quieter and I won't drive myself crazy. In an ideal world, I practice a full 2 hours in the afternoon. If I don't get a long, solid practice for myself on a fairly regular basis, it's not pretty. My body certainly needs that, but I also need it emotionally. Otherwise, I'm not good with people.

Speaking of people, I can't imagine teaching without practicing myself. How could I have anything useful to say? And how could I have that attitude of urgency, in the best sense of the word, that yoga is necessary? I certainly don't say that, but I think I exude that. *You must be here; it's essential.* That's the real message of yoga: this is your time to see who you are and how you are and recognize the attachments that keep getting in your way and examine your fears. There's a sense of urgency to that process and I think those of us who have our own practice know and feel and are not afraid. I don't have to say that out loud to my students because I live it so clearly and because my teaching is informed by my practice.

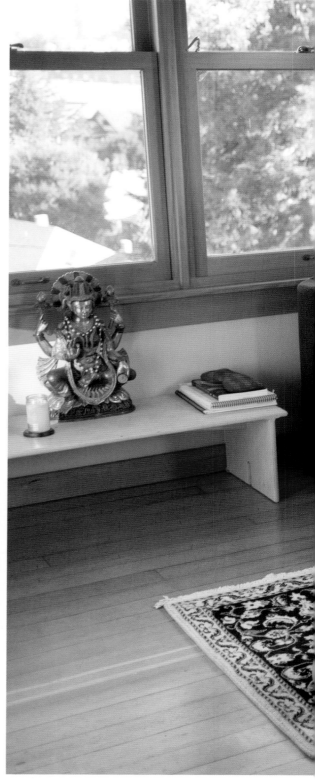

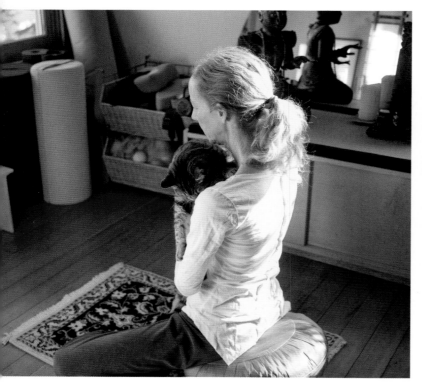

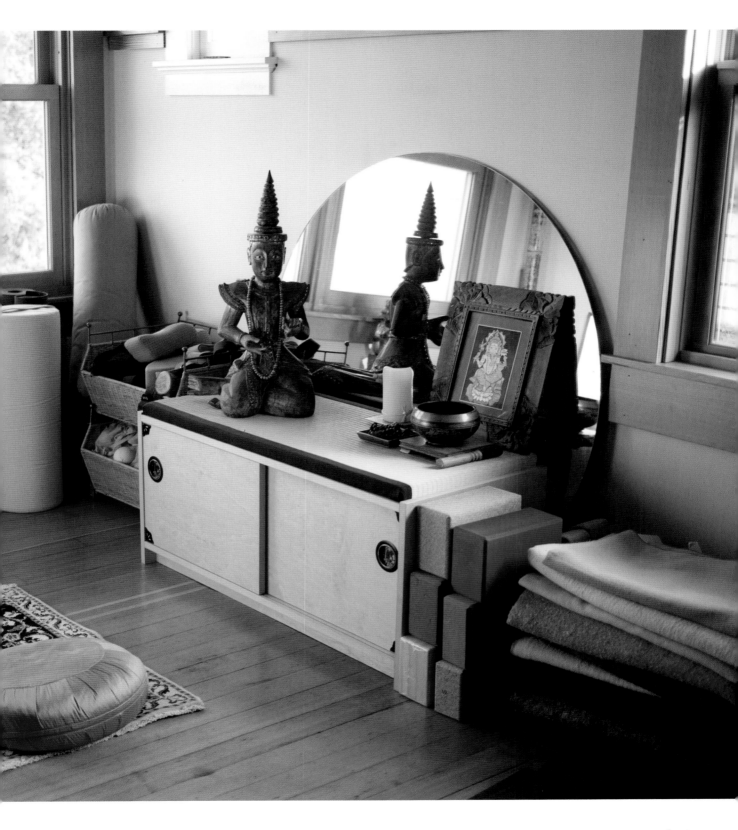

"The feeling of being deeply present in one's body is why we are all addicted to yoga."

KT Nelson

BERKELEY, CALIFORNIA | DANCE CHOREOGRAPHER

In addition to being artistic codirector of ODC/Dance in Oakland, KT is a dancer and an award-winning choreographer who mentors emerging artists in the Bay Area. She practices SmartFlow yoga with Annie Carpenter.

My home is a ninety-two-year-old Berkeley bungalow. There are two places in my house where I practice, one much more than the other. The dining room, which has always been used for making up dance movements and where my son used to practice the piano, is my main space. And because we don't heat our home, sometimes when it's cold I will practice in our tiny guest room. It's cozy, colorful, and filled with lots of books that I love.

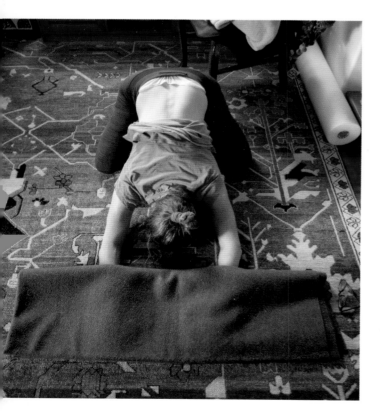

After dancing professionally for twenty-two years, it was yoga that shifted my love of dancing to my love of practicing. I found yoga to be the closest thing to performing. The concentration, the journey, the yielding to something larger than yourself, and the physical transformation of yoga all paralleled my experience of performing. Both experiences are ephemeral and difficult to put into words. I suppose the feeling of being deeply present in one's body is why we are all somewhat addicted to yoga.

I admit I've always been a goal-oriented person and now I am beginning to relax my agenda and just practice—20 minutes, 45 minutes, an hour, sometimes longer. This is a big deal for me. As an ex-dancer, I had some very specific notions about how much work I needed to do. Home practice was hard at first because I had a huge list of things I wanted to "accomplish." That word probably says it all. It would take me up to 3 hours, which of course made me very reluctant to get started!

I now love home practice because I don't have to go anywhere and I can spend time on areas where I need more work. I love Headstand and Shoulderstand and I can spend as much time in them as I want. Every once in a while I will get a correction in class and I will focus on that for six months or more. I still love taking classes because I can simply give myself over to whatever the particular sequencing is. That yielding is useful for me.

For the first ten years of my yoga practice, I was only doing yoga in class unless I was on the road and then I would practice in my hotel room. Then there was a moment back at home when I realized I was using yoga to counter stress in my life. One morning I was desperate to go to yoga class so I could handle my

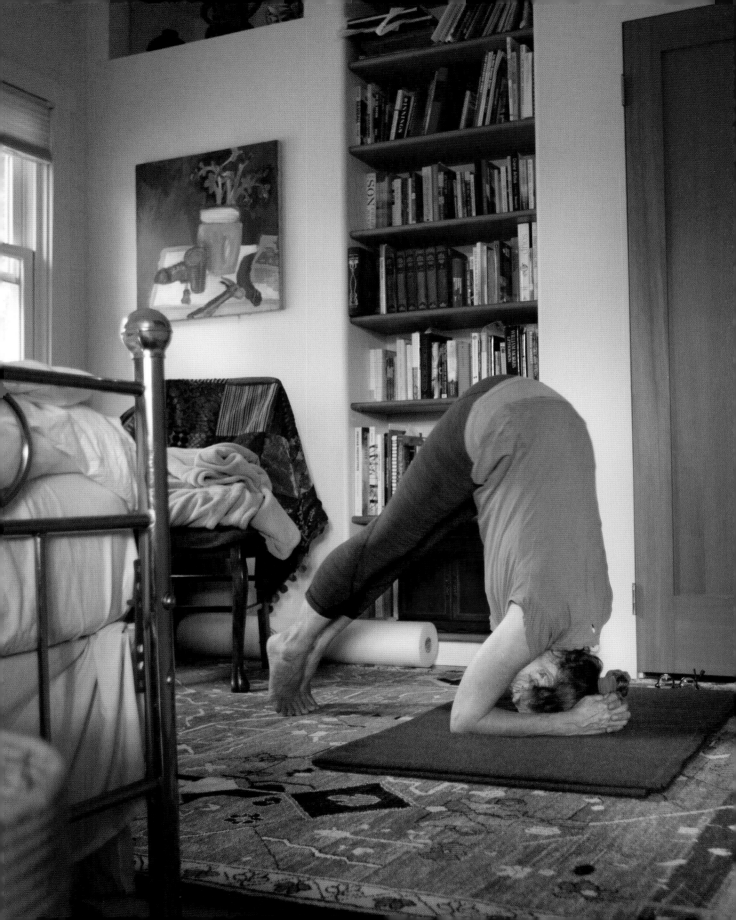

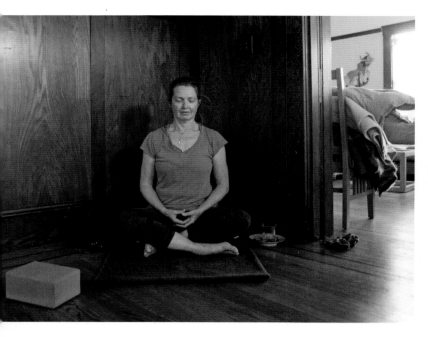

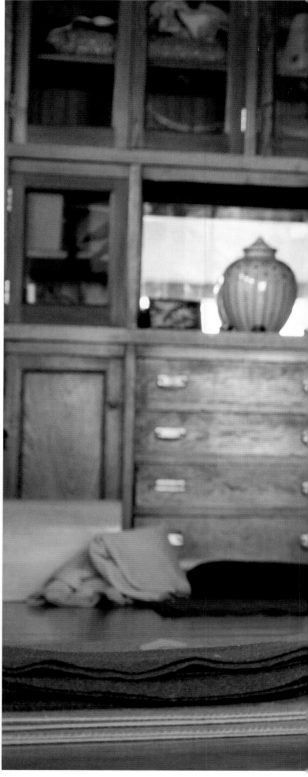

day at work. I realized how bad this was. I was not doing yoga to become aware or be present; I was doing it so I could go back into the harsh rat race and not feel so bad. I was using it like alcohol. That morning, I didn't go to class, but I sat down and thought about what I was doing. Since then, I have practiced yoga to know yoga.

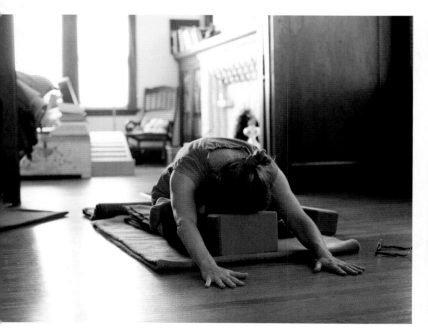

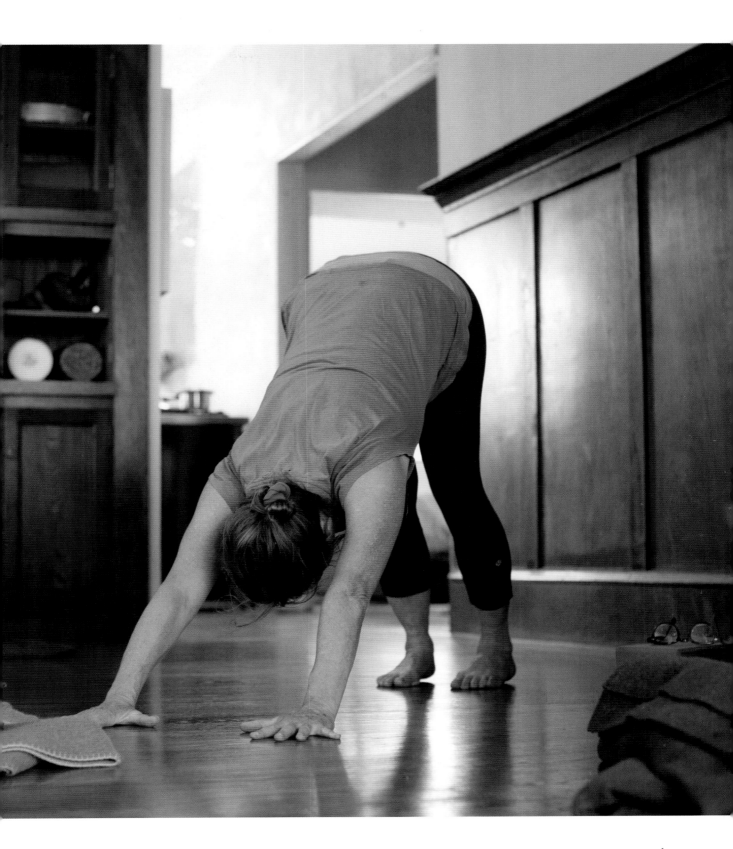

> *"All practices should be based in the endeavor to wake up from the delusion."*

Richard Freeman

BOULDER, COLORADO | YOGA TEACHER/YOGA STUDIO CO-OWNER

One of America's most beloved yoga teachers, Richard has the ability to weave various viewpoints into his teaching without losing the depth or integrity of any of them, which contributes to his unique, metaphorical teaching style.

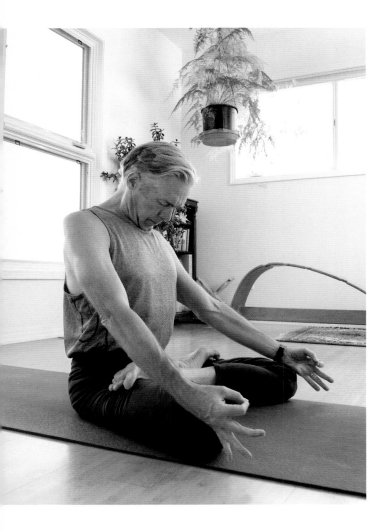

When we remodeled our house eleven years ago, we created two rooms exclusively for the practice of meditation and yoga. In both rooms we have small shrines with statues of our favorite deities and quite an assortment of sitting cushions, straps, bolsters, blankets, and strange experimental props that people have given us over the years. We also have a small library in each practice room that contains various scriptures, which we can read before or after practice. Because of this, we rarely do a complete practice any other place in the house, but we will often spontaneously do yoga poses in any room of the house, especially halfway up one of the staircases. The house is one big yoga prop.

Once you have an established practice, practicing alone allows you to concentrate more deeply and to fine-tune the alignment of the poses and the movement of the breath without reference to other practitioners or social norms and assumptions. For a beginning or intermediate practitioner, a solitary practice should be interspersed with practice with a teacher or a group of like-minded students so that you don't indulge your fantasies and delusional trips.

Your home practice can also be a meditation practice or a pranayama practice. Of course, you do meditation or pranayama *in* an asana, so you can't get away from it. All practices should be based in the endeavor to wake up from the delusion, which causes us to suffer, and when they are, this form of practice can make us compassionate and intelligent.

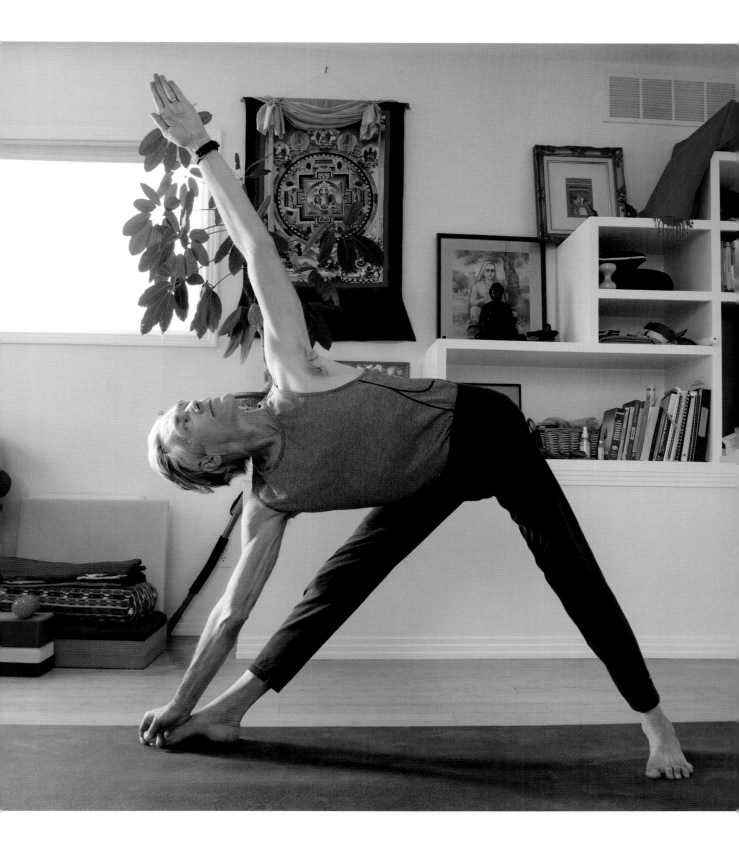

> *"I'm inspired by the kindness and admiration*
> *for others that yoga awakens within me."*

Mary Taylor

BOULDER, COLORADO | YOGA TEACHER/YOGA STUDIO CO-OWNER

Mary has practiced Ashtanga yoga since 1988, when she met Pattabhi Jois. Besides teaching yoga, Mary is on the faculty of Upaya Zen Center's Being with Dying program. She has a deep respect for the healing effects of yoga.

I find having a designated space in which to practice quite helpful. The space we've created has a still and open sense to it, so just walking into the room makes us *feel* different. I associate the room with the activities that go on there, and the meditative mindset that is cultivated through those activities. So when I walk in, even in a distracted state, I am immediately met with an appealing sense of calm. I'm invited to practice.

The room contains a statue of Ganesh and also a beautiful painting of the Medicine Buddha. Having sacred objects like these reminds us that our practice is actually in service of others. During a particularly difficult meditation practice—or in an asana that seems impossible—when my mind wanders into the realm of escape or grasping, sometimes just glancing at the altar or painting is enough to remind me to put everything back in context of the bigger picture of life. And that makes me smile at my silliness and also appreciate my own willingness to keep trying!

Having a defined space helps other family members, too. Whenever I have my mat rolled out or I'm sitting on my cushion, it's clear to anyone who passes

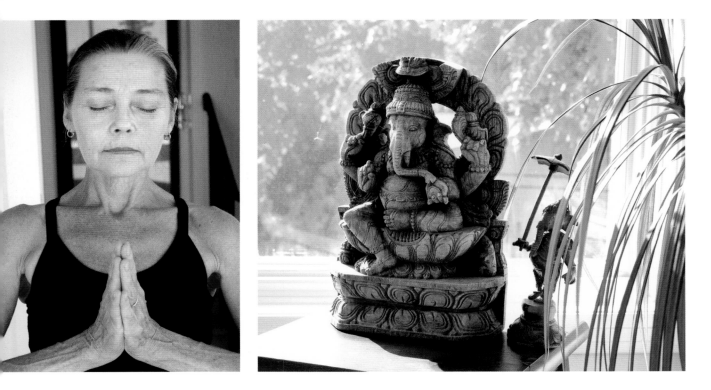

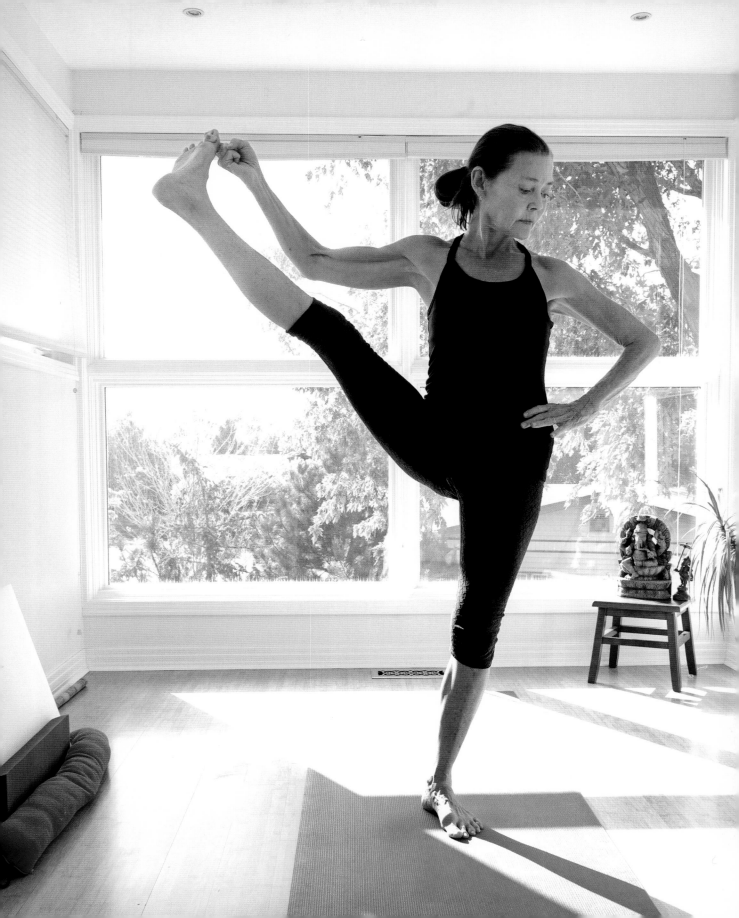

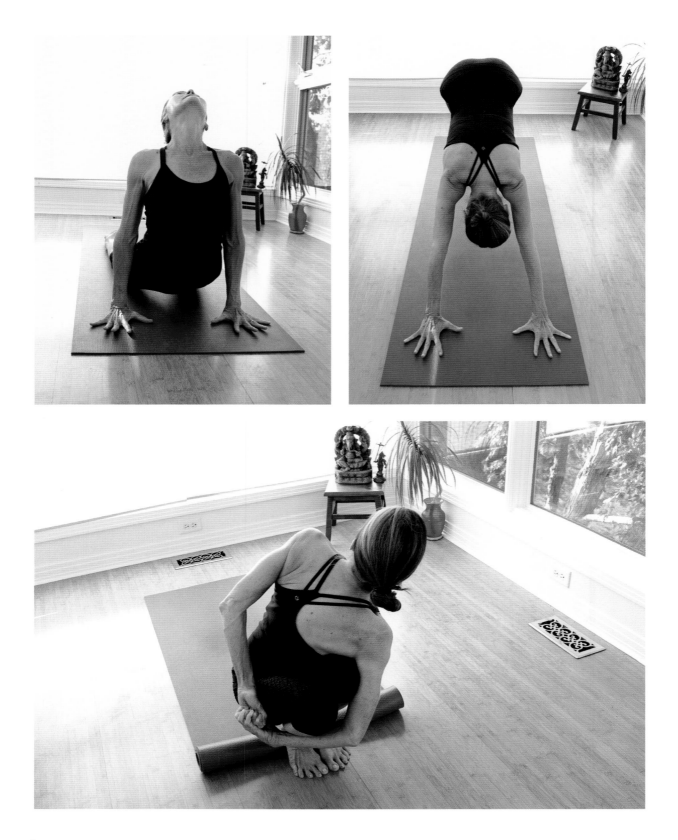

that I'm practicing—even our pets. It's not that I won't interact with others if they need something urgently, but they seem to pause before interrupting me. Even before I had the luxury of a room of my own, I would always practice in the same spot. I'd clean up all the toys strewn about the floor, fold back the carpet, and roll out my mat before closing the glass door to our back porch. It was clear I was practicing, but equally clear that if the need arose I could be interrupted. And chances were, because I'd been practicing, I would be in a good mood and not get annoyed at the interruption. Defining a place just for practice can remind you, as well as the others around you, that yoga and meditation are an integral part of your life that both nourish and nurture you deeply on an individual level.

I think what brings me back to the mat again and again is the feeling I have when it's over. Of course, some days the practice itself is wonderful, but some days it's pure torture. Mostly my mind is what tortures me, but even then or when I'm working my way around physical difficulties, I can honestly say that almost one hundred percent of the time, if I just stick with it and do a full practice, I'll feel better. Having practiced pretty much every day for more than thirty years, the struggle to stay on the mat is really not so much a part of things anymore. In the beginning, however, I'd sometimes resist. So I'd make a deal with myself to just do three Sun Salutations. Nine times out of ten, after a couple of those I'd think, "Well, I'll just do a few standing poses." And before I knew it, I had done a complete practice. I also used to make a bargain with myself—I could do a short practice *if* I did the poses I hated (which in the beginning were plentiful). Somehow I realized early on that my mind wanted me to skip the things I found difficult, and I felt that it was important to not do that—at least on the yoga mat.

More than any other form, a self-practice reveals all levels of mind that arise. It immediately becomes clear (sometimes painfully) that all of the interruptions are your own—thoughts, physical sensations, emotions, excuses, interpretations, judgments, wanderings of mind, disciplines of mind, and on and on. Self-practice can make you feel embarrassed at how petty your own mind can be, or astonished at the vastness of your breath or the depths of your heart. (And both of those insights can come in one practice, if not one breath cycle!) My self-practice is where I really

MARY'S PRACTICE ADVICE

- Be patient with yourself. Notice what you feel before, during, and after the practice. Give it time and don't give up—the benefits of your practice (for yourself and for others) come slowly and after a long period of uninterrupted practice. But if you miss a day, don't worry.

- By simply paying attention to the thoughts, feelings, and sensations that arise, you'll soon discern the appropriate rhythm of your practice. Watch for patterns of avoidance, rigidity, or laziness. Notice as clearly as you can, and start over again and again. Remember that 5 minutes on the mat is a million times better than no practice at all. Your practice may soon expand if you stay patient, open, and curious.

feel connected and where I feel the thread of internal awareness that I love so much.

I'm inspired by the kindness, tolerance, compassion, and true admiration for others that yoga awakens within me. After practice I feel deeply connected to and moved by others. I also feel more clearheaded. No matter how "good" or "bad" my practice was, I simply feel better and more tuned in to my environment and to others. I wouldn't trade that for anything.

Home practice can be just sitting, chanting, meditating, or pranayama. But in my experience, the grounding that well-defined, specific practices provide is essential for keeping the mind clear and focused. One way to differentiate a practice from your everyday activities is that a practice has a defined form, and when you begin, you set the intention to practice (often by offering a chant or simply drawing the mind inside) and then again and again during the practice you bring your attention back to the intention you've set at the beginning. When the practice is over, it is also helpful to recognize that it has ended by chanting or taking a moment to reflect internally.

> *"Yoga is a gift that we have in this life. We must use it to gain wisdom and knowledge."*

Sonny Rollins

WOODSTOCK, NEW YORK | AWARD-WINNING SAXOPHONE PLAYER

One of the world's most influential jazz musicians, tenor saxophonist Sonny credits his meditation and yoga practice with his longevity and his ability to see the world with pure joy and understanding.

I have been performing as a musician forever. Back in the early 1950s, I became interested in the metaphysical and in Buddhism and yoga. I started yoga by reading Swami Sivananda's books and tried to figure it all out on my own. Finally, in 1967, I went to India, near Bombay, where I studied with Chinmayananda, a disciple of Swami Sivananda. Chinmayananda told me that my yoga practice should be karma yoga—the yoga of service. No expectations of reciprocity. How could I do that as a professional musician? Music is a very competitive business. But I finally came to understand that I really couldn't worry about how famous or popular I was. My soul must progress through its journeys.

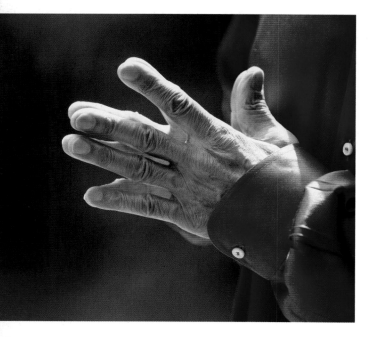

Since then, yoga has become a part of me, integrated deeply into my life. When I began asanas I was transported to such tranquility that I could forget the worries of the world. Yoga allows me to meld higher forces with the body—body going to the mind; body going to the spirit. I am good where I am right now, so grateful for my practice. It shows me that the world is the little picture; the spirit is the big picture. I'm happy now. I'm grateful to have come to this point in my life where I have more understanding of what life is all about. I am always praying, always giving thanks. I don't necessarily pray to someone up there; we are God, we are already Divine Essence, so don't sweat it!

As time wore on, my body got a little cranky, so I don't do much asana anymore—just the basic stuff. For some years now my practice has focused on *bhakti* (devotion), *raja* (using the energy of the mind), and *dhyana* (meditation). But any yoga I do can immediately put me in a spiritual frame of mind. I still meditate. I pray. I can drop into the spiritual realm anywhere. Yoga is a gift that we have in this life. We must use it to gain wisdom and knowledge, to move us toward a deeper understanding of ourselves and of the world.

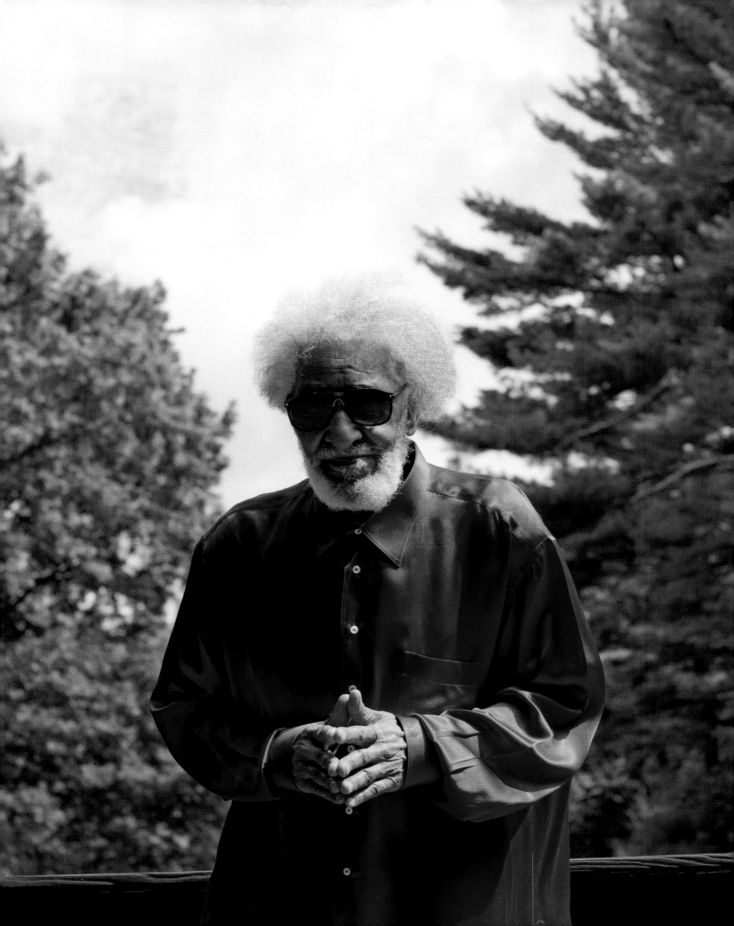

"We practice so that, ultimately, nothing can knock us off the center of our day."

Tias Little

SANTA FE, NEW MEXICO | YOGA TEACHER/YOGA STUDIO OWNER

Tias and his wife Surya created Prajna Yoga, a profound journey inward. Through yoga poses, dharma study, guided meditation, the yoga of sound, and somatic awareness, their practice allows for unique, personal transformation.

My wife Surya and I built our dream practice space, from the ground up, on our ten-acre parcel of land outside Santa Fe. Built by a yogi carpenter, Robert LaPorte, and designed by his wife, Paula Baker, our home studio complements and enhances the mindfulness of the yoga experience. They used nontoxic materials and natural finishes and the mud walls are made of straw clay. In building our practice space, we wanted to create a living structure that amplifies, not detracts from, the prana within the practice space.

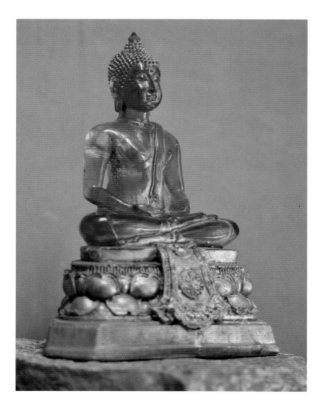

TIAS'S SAMPLE PRACTICE

- Supta Padangusthasana II (Reclining Hand-to-Big-Toe Pose), supporting outside leg with a block or bolster

- Anantasana (Sleeping Vishnu Pose)

- Supta Dandasana (Reclining Staff Pose), back on floor, both legs extending upward

- Adho Mukha Svanasana (Downward-Facing Dog), with head supported

- Prasarita Padottanasana (Wide-Angle Standing Forward Bend), with head supported

- Utthita Trikonasana (Extended Triangle Pose)

- Utthita Parsvakonasana (Extended Side Angle Pose)

- Virabhadrasana II (Warrior II Pose)

- Ardha Chandrasana (Half-Moon Pose)

- Upavishta Konasana (Wide-Angle Seated Forward Bend), with head supported

- Seated meditation

- Savasana (Corpse Pose)

The studio has unique windows, situated to allow a glimpse of the natural world outdoors. Within the space, we've placed elements that remind us of the raw, nonlinear beauty of nature—a gnarled juniper bough, black river stones, irregular pieces of sandstone

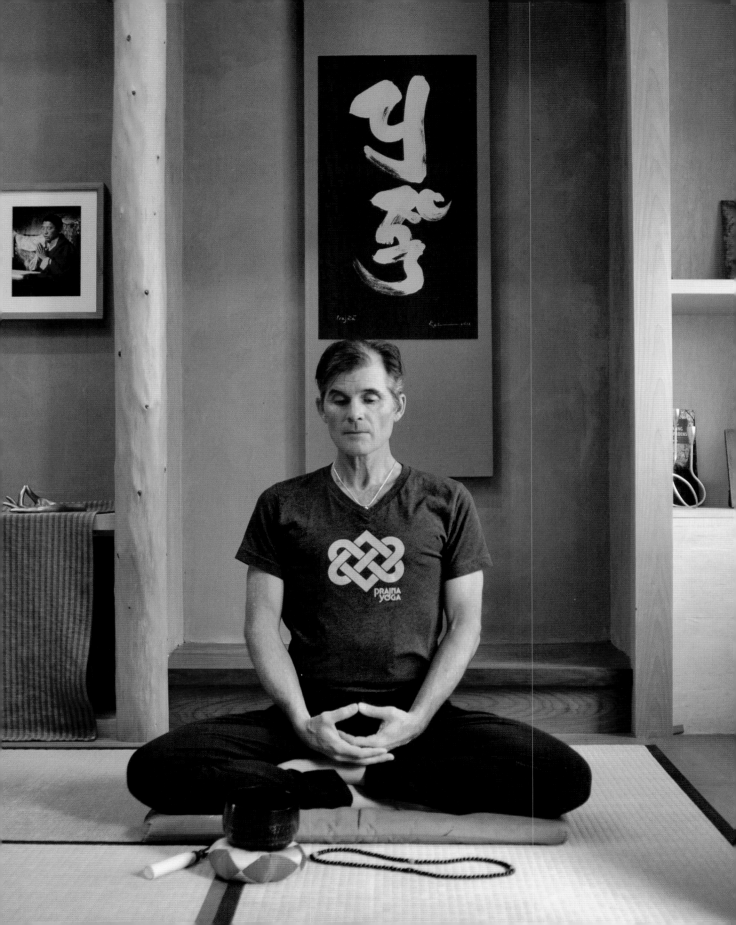

moss rock. Like Zen temples in Japan, where a spare and pleasing aesthetic inspires the mind to go still, our practice space elicits deep calm.

I always do home practice. I don't like to leave my home until I commune with my inner guides, allies, and angels. When I do not yoke to the presence of the spirit inside and breathe life into my pranic sheath, then I am prone to distraction, irritation, or carelessness throughout the day. The pressures of the world and the demands of people tend to wither the pranic sheath. When our prana is depleted and our vitality is weakened, one is prone to disease of all kinds. The practice provides not only a physical buffer, but also a kind of psychic shield. We practice so that, ultimately, nothing can knock us off the center of our day.

I am a morning practitioner. I get up, take a pee, and go right to the meditation cushion in my practice space. Meditation is a critical adjunct to asana. Meditation is really the backbone of a yoga practice. It allows for the Pause, a short series of moments when we are not required to do anything. The Pause is an invitation to reside in silence and stillness. In my experience, the more penetrating the Pause, the more I begin to heal my neurotic self. Sitting in an open and relaxed posture allows for healing on a subliminal level, a cellular level. The Pause expands our sense of time and space, both heart space and mind space.

The most auspicious time to sit is the threshold time between night and day and dream and waking. This is when I am most permeable and open to the small voice

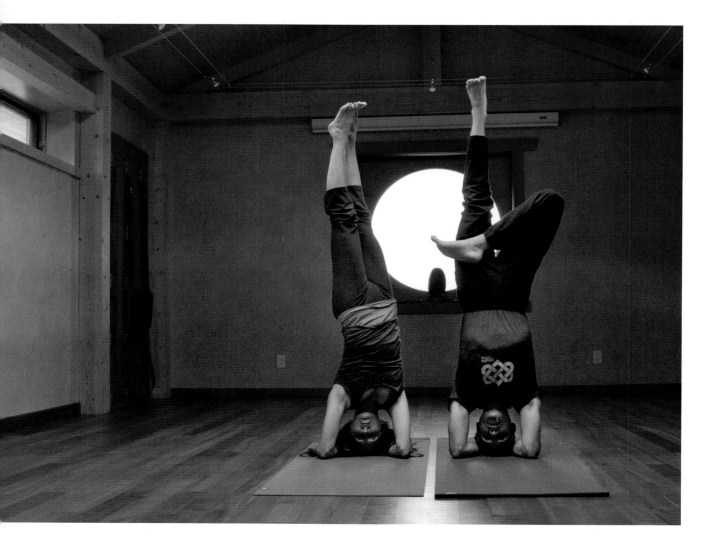

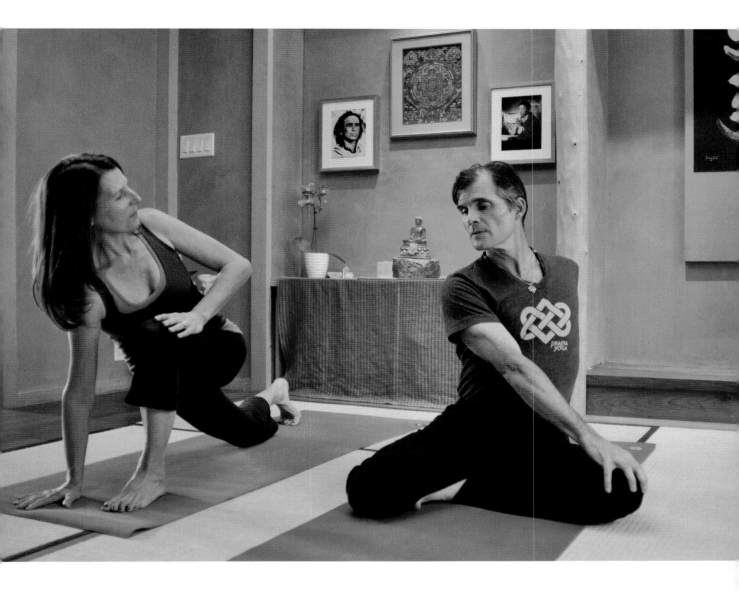

of the Unspeakable Spirit that dwells within. This is the time before the recycling truck goes barreling down the road and the neighbors take their morning walks, yapping on their cell phones. This is a time when my pulses are soft, my heart rate is slow, and my mind is a little bit empty. In morning meditation, I track my dreams. After twenty-five years of doing yoga, much of my practice is focused on the subtle (and not-so-subtle) churnings of my depth psyche. Impressions of fear, shame, and pride bubble up in the dreamtime. By sitting with the afterimages of dreams, I catch glimpses of my shadow. Early morning practice is best for being with the outlines of the shadows that surface in dreams.

For me, it is paramount to ride the changing edge of being, for I am always in a state of becoming, never static. Thus, the practice should never simply be routine. For instance, I started in Ashtanga vinyasa yoga when I was in my early twenties. Now that I am over the age of fifty, I do a very different practice than I did twenty years ago. I believe the practice should always stay fresh, creative, and interesting. It is only "routine" in that discipline and consistency are required to step onto the mat every day. However, as we age we must skillfully conform our practice to be in accord with the changes that happen in our bodies, minds, and spirits. In this sense, the practice should always be evolving.

> *"Showing up in any way is always better than not showing up at all."*

Anna Guest-Jelly

NASHVILLE, TENNESSEE | YOGA TEACHER

Founder and CEO (Curvy Executive Officer) of Curvy Yoga, a training and inspiration portal for yogis of all shapes and sizes, Anna encourages anyone wanting a body-positive practice that supports them to "grab life by the curves."

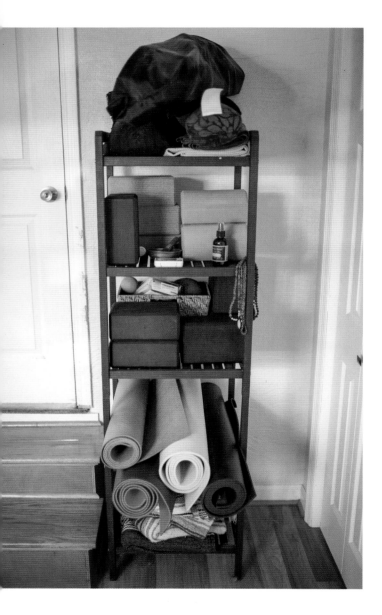

Coziness is my top priority for my home yoga space. I want to be in a space where I feel nourished and where I can drop into my practice at any time. My space doubles as my office and the laundry room, so it's not that I have this luxurious, exclusive space. The primary way I make my space sacred is by deeming it so. Finding my practice even when my computer is three feet in front of me and my laundry is on the floor waiting to be washed is what it's all about for me. I love practicing here; it's the perfect intersection of the practical and the spiritual, which is exactly how I view my practice—concrete and transcendent.

My biggest challenge is that I tell myself I'm too busy. Notice I didn't say I *am* too busy. Like most people, I very well may be, but the true challenge is all the internal drama I stir up around it in addition to the actual things that need to be done. A friend of mine, Andrea Scher, once shared that she was

ANNA'S PRACTICE ADVICE

- Life is ebb and flow. Life is change. And when we fight life, we find resistance, which makes it easier to give up. Your yoga practice may never be that perfect thing you wish it to be. And that's OK.

- If you're prepared to roll with what each day brings, it's entirely possible to create a consistent home yoga practice. The key is knowing that consistent is not the same as homogeneous.

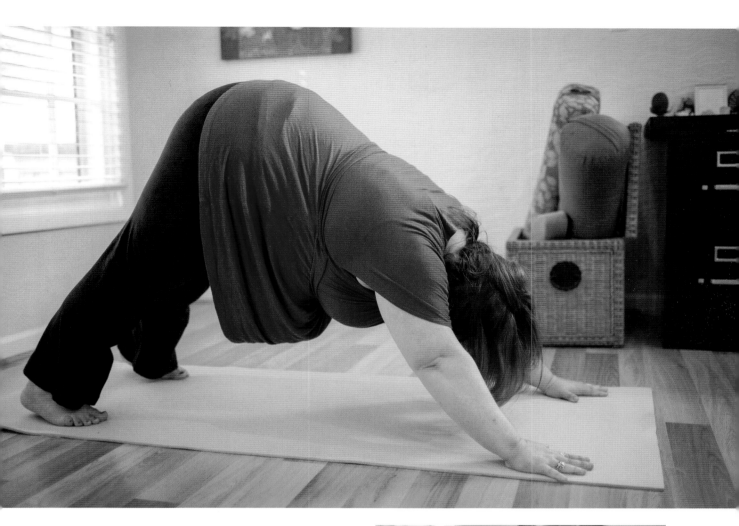

experimenting with a mantra of "I'm actually not that busy." When I came across that, I decided to try it, too, and I was shocked at what a difference it makes. When I can loosen the fear and panic I create around time, it's amazing what opens up—without my to-do list changing at all.

I'm constantly abandoning myself, either by checking out or focusing on hurtful thoughts from my inner critic. My home practice is what brings me back, time and again, because it's very "no muss, no fuss." I don't even have to change clothes if that feels like too much of an obstacle on any given day. Showing up in any way is always better than not showing up at all. My practice is a connection with and acceptance of my body and self, which then fills my tank so that I can give to others.

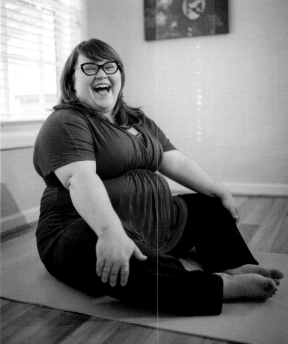

"Unexpected things happen to cause you to miss your practice and that is where yoga is."

Jaclyn Roberson

COLORADO SPRINGS, COLORADO | YOGA TEACHER/CHEMISTRY PROFESSOR

Jaclyn began her formal yoga training at Shoshoni Yoga Ashram, a rich lineage that focuses on the cultivation of inner peace through ancient yogic teachings by surrendering into an open mind and an open heart.

As a mom, yoga has helped me to be patient. A regular meditation practice helps me to surrender expectations, to cultivate deeper love and devotion, and to connect with the *seva* (service) of daily life. Attending class is a nice escape and provides valuable personal time, but surrendering to the present is so much more of the practice. Unexpected things happen that cause you to miss your practice or disrupt your meditation and that is where yoga is—being able to surrender in the moment with a loving heart.

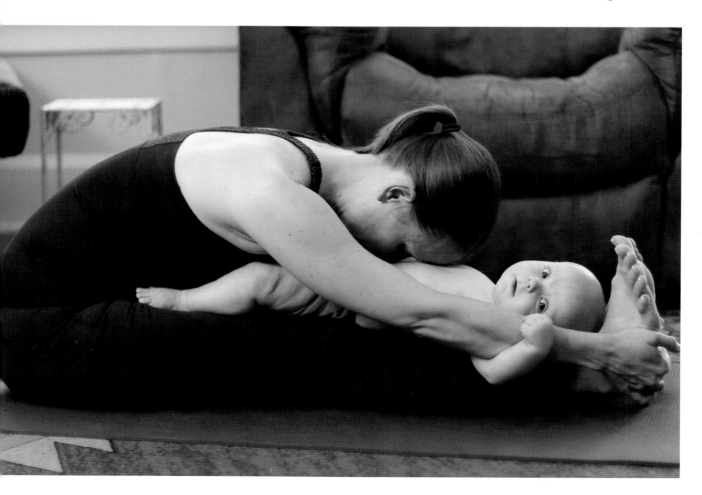

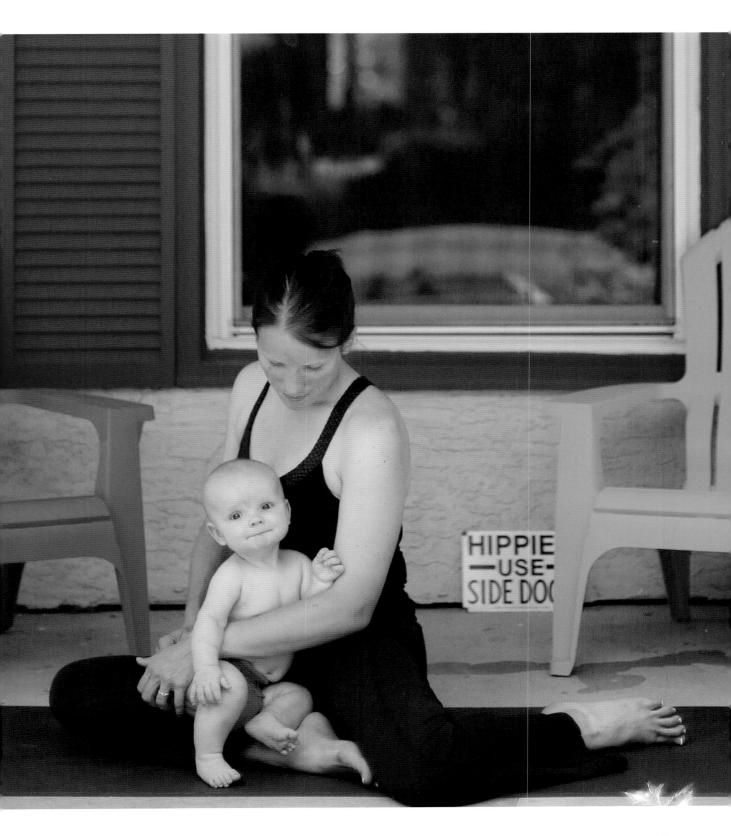

"The creative process is doing things that you aren't supposed to do. Be as free as possible."

Angela Farmer & Victor Van Kooten

LESBOS, GREECE | YOGA TEACHERS/YOGA STUDIO CO-OWNERS

Angela and Victor encourage their students to begin an internal exploration that is both deeply experiential and delightfully playful, a process that guides them to greater freedom and the joy of discovering their own personal practices.

You can learn by observing many different things. In our place in Lesbos, Greece, Angela has the particular habit of feeding all of the cats that wander by. It's such fun to see the characters. We feed the cats and the cats feed us. We have too little time to do nothing or to be bored.

And we like each other a lot. You can have a lot of love and a relationship doesn't have to become stuck. Yoga helps. Look at yourself; listen to yourself. And really look at each other, too.

ANGELA: It has been through my yoga practice that I've come to listen internally to myself. It used to be that I was out to prove something, to improve and

VICTOR'S PRACTICE ADVICE

❁ Doubt as much as possible. See what is true and what is not true for you. You come to your own path and your own personal yoga practice.

❁ My advice is to be curious and objective. The creative process is doing things that you aren't supposed to do. Experiment. Be as free as possible. Get interested in the space inside you. Do quiet listening.

ANGELA'S PRACTICE ADVICE

❁ Instead of doing a routine, just sit and slowly go forward. It could be in any stretch, but notice the parts of the body that are not connecting with the ground. Feel the ground supporting you.

❁ When your body resists, watch the tiny places where you have a fraction of resistance. Wait and listen. See how long it takes to release and go further. That is the beginning of self-trust.

challenge, and to do better asana—and battle with myself and beat myself up to get somewhere. I used to have a strict-training type of yoga, but it isn't about that anymore. A shift happened for me about thirty years ago, and I started to listen to my inner energy. It was an unknown path. But I learned that each part of the body has a voice. And trauma is hidden, especially in places that have been hiding and don't want to be seen. If I can be gentle with those places and communicate with them, they slowly shift and change and open up.

So now I'm exploring and unfolding rather than going out and trying to achieve something. I'm more tolerant and mentally flexible. I have more focus and

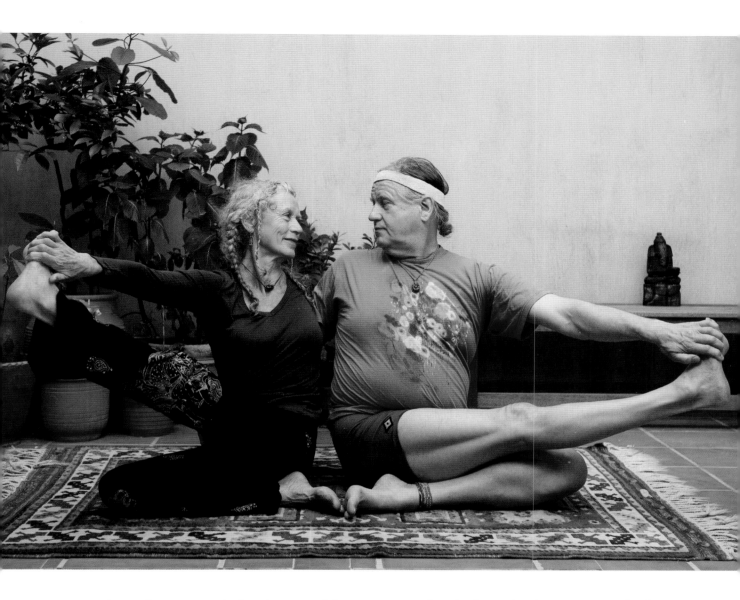

more patience. I respect my body a lot more. I let myself sleep more when I need to. I eat, play, and have more inner joy. I follow the young kid of eight who lives inside me. She gets to swim in the wintertime. She gets to play plenty.

VICTOR: As I get older, I go beyond the body and connect with the sky and the ground. I'm more patient with myself. I used to be tough on myself in my practice, but I've learned to be receptive to the feminine side. Rather than doing, I try to open up. Once you are more receptive, you realize that even little things are as important as big things.

We humans take for granted that life is this way or that way. Parents, teachers, and voices tell us we are supposed to live life a certain way. But I've learned I need to listen to myself and rethink everything I was trained to do. It's undoing.

"The gift of yoga is its connection to the body, which leads to a connection to the soul."

Maria Rodale

EMMAUS, PENNSYLVANIA | PUBLISHER/AUTHOR/ACTIVIST

A passionate advocate on behalf of organic gardening and farming, Maria is also an author, editor, and the CEO and chair of Rodale, Inc., the world's leading multimedia publishing company focusing on health, wellness, and the environment.

Doing yoga at home means I don't compare myself to any others and I can be present to what is. The most consistent, reliable way for me to do that is to have a teacher come to my house.

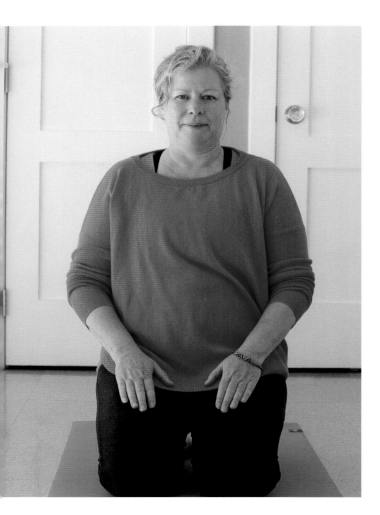

MARIA'S PRACTICE ADVICE

- You need a teacher because a teacher can customize a practice for you, but you also need to get over the fear of doing things wrong when you're on your own.

- Don't take yoga too seriously. It's simply a part of a whole way of living without rigidity.

When I moved into my new house, I wanted to create a room just for yoga. I didn't want to move furniture or rearrange anything to practice. The room has windows and doors on both sides, so it has a wonderful indoor/outdoor feel to it. When I do asana with a teacher—ideally twice a week—we are together for about 2 hours. My three daughters often join in, so lots of talking and laughing go on, along with a nice, long sequence.

I approach yoga as a way of being, not just a physical practice. I do a lot of spiritual reading on my own. My most recent area of study—over the last two years or so—is shamanism. I need to do that inner work and discovery so that I have the vision and energy to do the work that I do out in the world.

Listening to my body keeps me coming back to yoga. I need to be in my body. The gift of yoga is its connection to the body, which leads to a connection to the soul. Yoga makes us hyperaware of the senses and the energy around us.

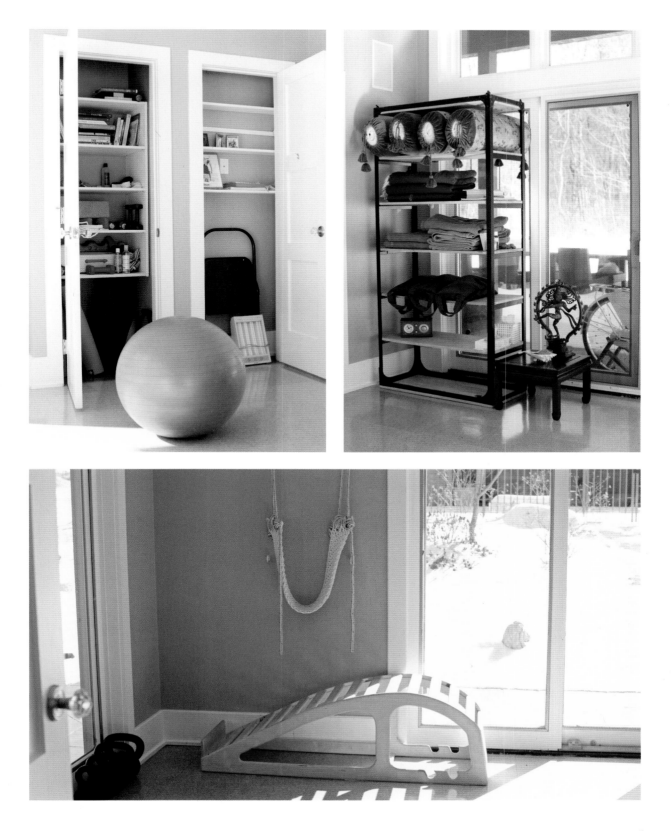

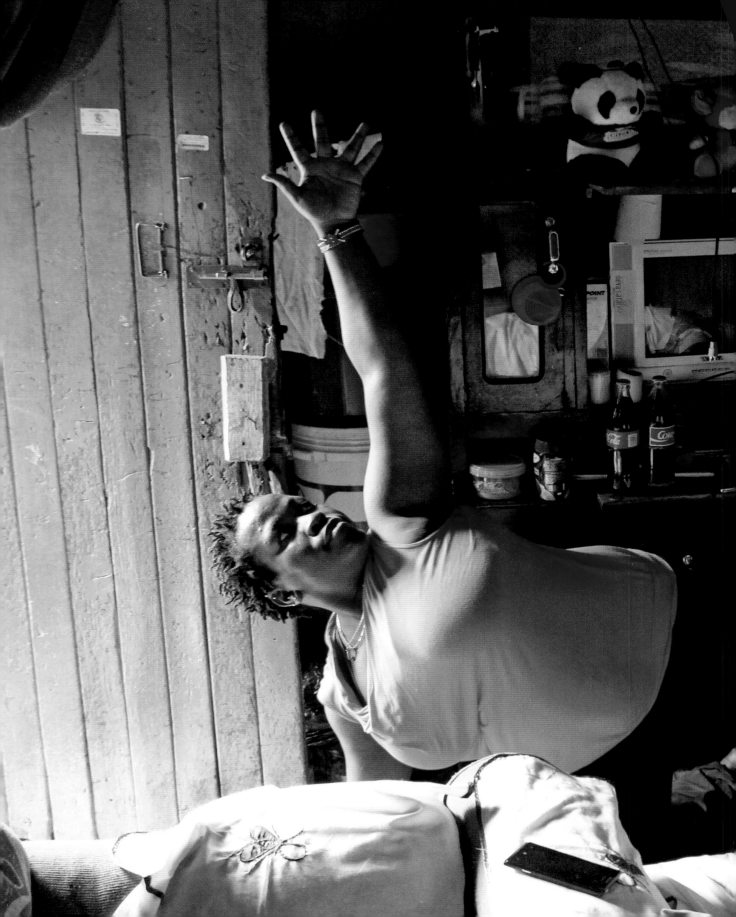

"In my home practice, I like to warm up with Sun Salutations and then I work on poses that I find challenging, like handstands and a number of binding poses.

Some of my students are deaf and blind and some have cerebral palsy. I feel so inspired by the strength and connection of my community and by sharing my work with those students with special needs."

Magdaline Adhiambo

NAIROBI, KENYA | YOGA TEACHER

The Magic 10

SHARON GANNON

I'm on the go so much that I needed a practice that was doable, one that could also prepare me for a longer practice, like my meditation practice. I've been doing it for about fifteen years now. There are ten pretty simple asanas that anyone can do—in 10 minutes or less. Of course, you can modify if you need to.

1. Adho Mukha Svanasana
   (Downward-Facing Dog)
   10 breaths
2. Uttanasana (Standing Forward Bend)
   10 breaths
3. Malasana
   (Garland Pose)
   10 breaths
4. Teepee Twist
   5 breaths each side
5. Ardha Matsyendrasana
   (Half Lord of the Fishes Pose)
   5 breaths each side
6. Ardha Purvottanasana
   (Half Upward Plank Pose)
   10 breaths
7. Adho Mukha Vrksasana (Handstand)
   25 breaths
8. Tadasana (Mountain Pose) variation
   4 breaths
9. Parsva Urdhva Hastasana
   (Side-Bending Upward Salute)
   1 breath each side 4 times
10. Spinal Rolls (see following spread)
    12 to 16 breaths

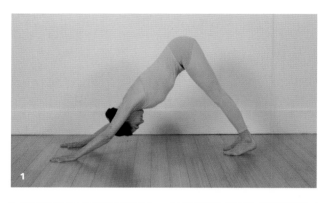

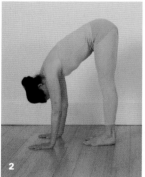

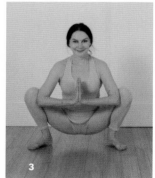

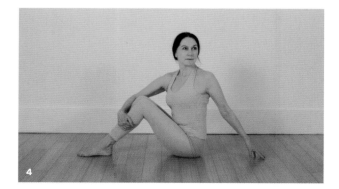

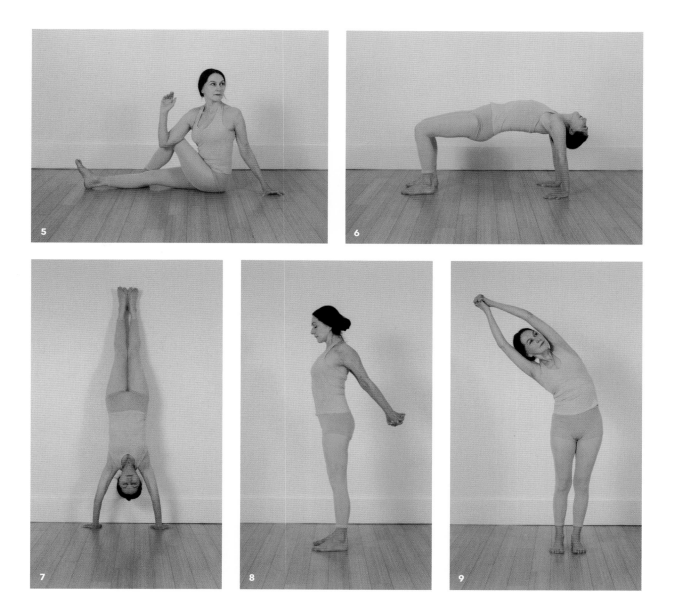

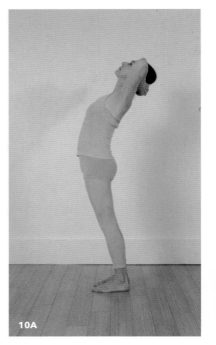

10A

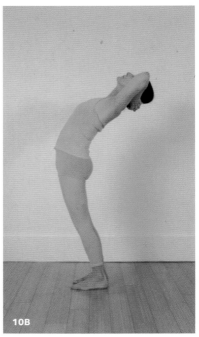

10B

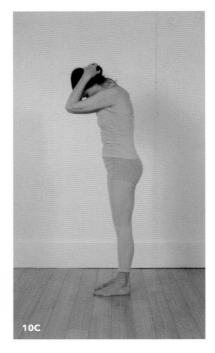

10C

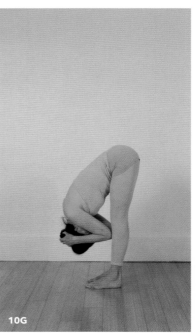

10G

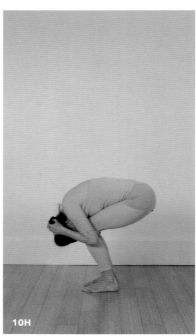

10H

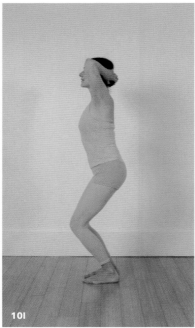

10I

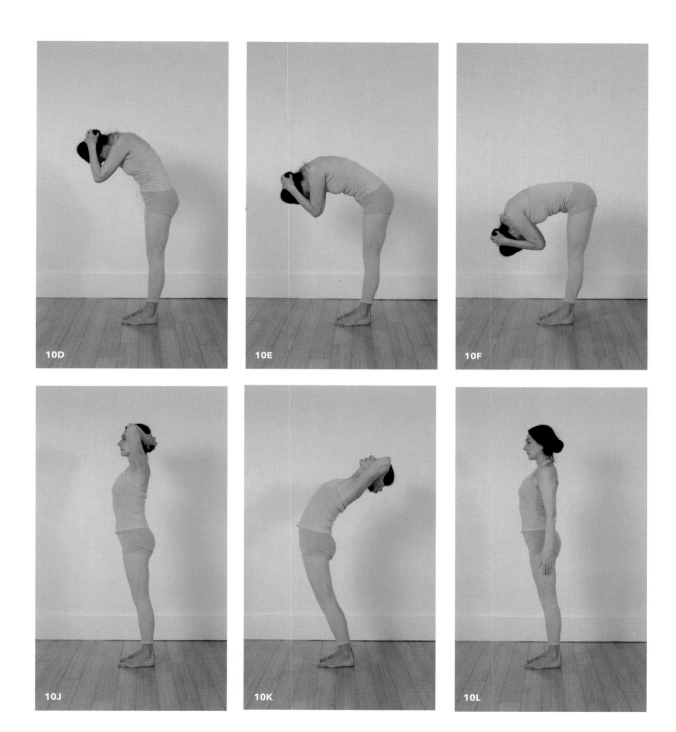

Ease into Urdhva Dhanurasana

JASON CRANDELL

This sequence prepares you for Wheel Pose by opening the shoulders and upper back as well as the front sheath of the body—specifically the quadriceps and hip flexors. It also builds heat in the whole body. All of this should help you feel more ease, more space, more joy in your backbend. Instead of focusing on going deep, focus on creating evenness. When you practice this way, not only will the pose feel a whole lot better, you'll be more apt to open the places that need it and derive the overall benefits of backbending.

WARM-UPS: Before you dive into the sequence, take a few minutes in seated meditation; from there, move into the first pose—Urdhva Baddha Hastasana in Vajrasana (Bound Hand Thunderbolt Pose). Hold each pose for 3 to 5 breaths.

1. Urdhva Baddha Hastasana in Vajrasana (Bound Hand Thunderbolt Pose)
2. Adho Mukha Svanasana (Downward-Facing Dog)
3. Anjaneyasana (Low Lunge)
   From Downward-Facing Dog, bring your left foot forward between your hands, back knee down.
4. Anjaneyasana (Low Lunge) Twist
   From Anjaneyasana, reach around and take hold of your back foot with your left hand. Unwind, lift your back knee, and come into . . .
5. High Lunge
6. High Lunge Twist
   From High Lunge, exhale your hands to prayer and twist to the left. Release the twist and move into . . .
7. Virabhadrasana I (Warrior I)
   Return to Downward-Facing Dog

Repeat poses 3 through 7 on the other side.

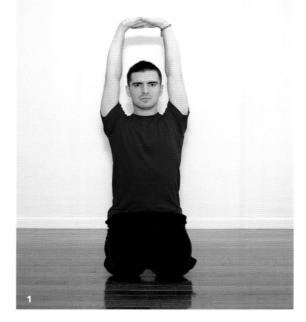

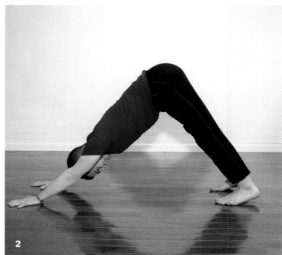

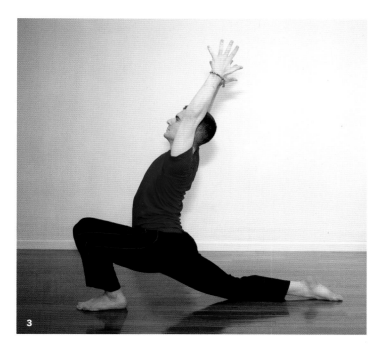

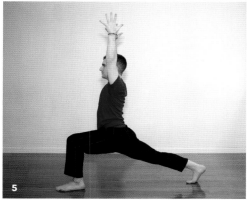

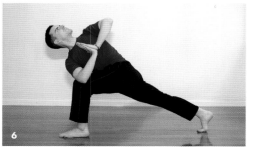

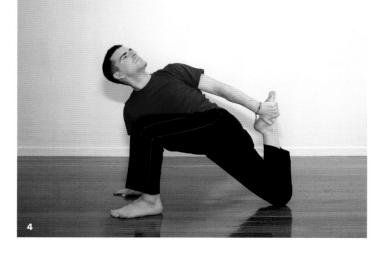

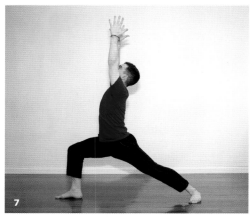

8. Adho Mukha Svanasana
   (Downward-Facing Dog) wall variation
9. Adho Mukha Vrksasana (Handstand)
   at the wall
10. Pincha Mayurasana
    (Feathered Peacock Pose) at the wall
11. Balasana (Child's Pose)
    Hold for several breaths.
12. Ardha Matsyendrasana
    (Half Lord of the Fishes Pose)
    Hold for 3 to 5 breaths and repeat on
    the other side.
13. Salabhasana (Locust Pose)
    Hold for 3 to 5 breaths and release your
    forehead to the floor.
14. Bhujangasana (Cobra Pose)
    Release your forehead to the floor and
    roll over onto your back for . . .
15. Setu Bandha Sarvangasana
    (Bridge Pose)
    Hold for 5 breaths or longer.
16. Urdhva Dhanurasana (Full Wheel)
    Stay in the pose for as long as you can
    maintain the proper alignment.

FINISHING POSES: End your practice with
Supta Padangusthasana (Reclined Hand-
to-Big-Toe Pose), followed by Apanasana
(Knees-to-Chest Pose), and a simple reclined
twist of your choice. And, don't forget
Savasana (Corpse Pose)!

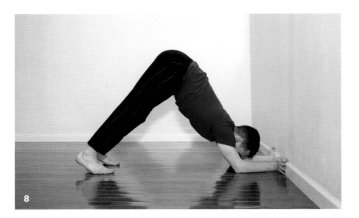

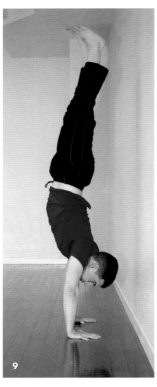

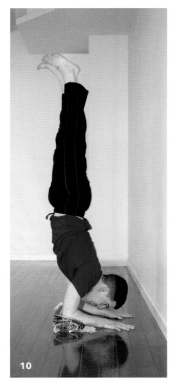

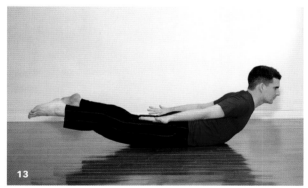

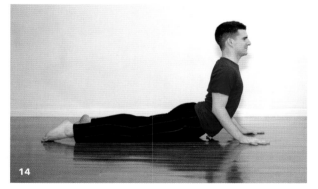

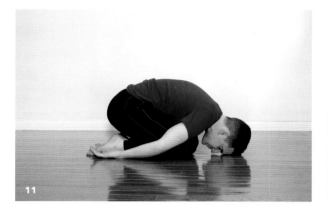

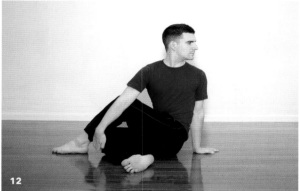

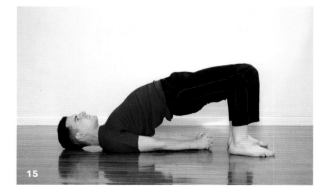

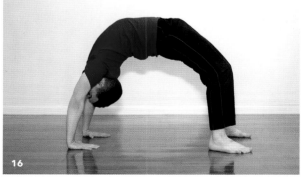

From Effort to Joy

CYNDI LEE

This short home practice sequence cultivates three important aspects of yoga: *tapas*
(practice or simplicity), *svadhyaya* (self-study),
and *ishvara pranidhana* (surrender). Tapas helps
you focus on your own practice, your own body,
instead of worrying about what else needs to get
done or what other people are up to. Svadhyaya
calls for a healthy dose of openheartedness,
humor, and a sense of adventure, and ishvara
pranidhana reminds you that it's not about getting somewhere; it's about the journey.

WARM-UPS: Begin with a few seated stretches or
a nice, long Downward-Facing Dog.

Practice this entire sequence on one side before
doing the other. Hold each pose for 3 to 5 breaths.

1. Utkatasana (Chair Pose)
2. Utkatasana variation (Ankle-to-Knee Pose)
    Cross your left ankle just above your right
    knee and flex your left foot. Unwind into . . .
3. Virabhadrasana I (Warrior I)
    . . . in a mild backbend and open to . . .
4. Virabhadrasana II (Warrior II)
    Straighten the front leg and inhale to . . .
5. Viparita Trikonasana (Reverse Triangle Pose)
    Cartwheel your hands to the floor,
    moving into . . .
6. High Lunge
    Step back to . . .
7. Adho Mukha Svanasana split
    (Three-Legged Downward-Facing Dog)
    Thread top leg under and through into . . .
8. Adho Mukha Parivṛtta Trikonasana
    (Downward-Facing Twisted Triangle Pose)
    Rewind that action and return to . . .
9. High Lunge
    Straighten your front leg and walk to . . .

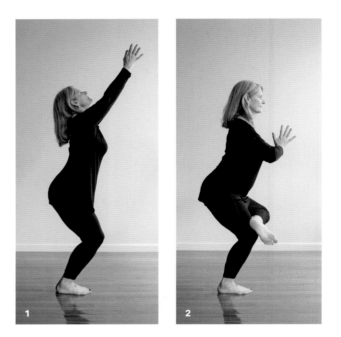

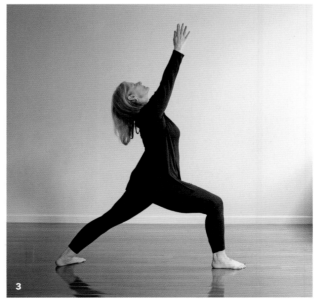

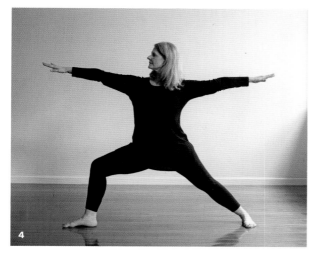

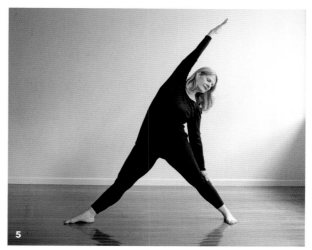

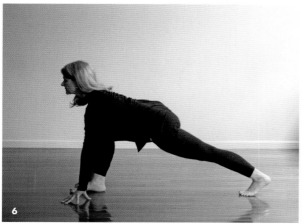

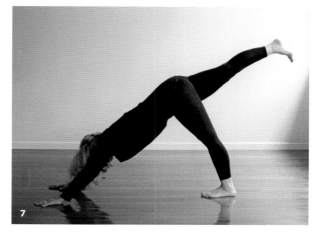

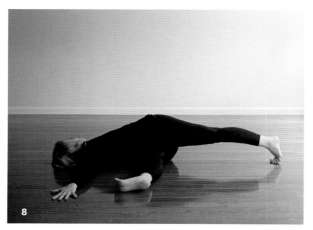

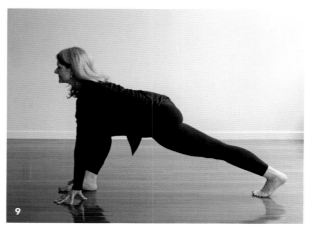

10. Prasarita Padottanasana
    (Wide-Legged Standing Forward Bend)
    Either stay here, or, if your head can reach the
    floor, do a Headstand before coming into . . .

11. Parivrtta Prasarita Padottanasana
    (Twisted Wide-Legged Standing
    Forward Bend)
    Walk around to your front leg and
    come into . . .

12. Eka Pada Rajakapotanasana (Pigeon Pose)
    Bending your back leg, hold on to it so
    you feel as if you are on the front of a ship.
    Swing your back leg around and place it on
    top of your front leg and move into . . .

13. Parivrtta Agnistambhasana
    (Twisted Fire Log Pose)
    Come out of the twist. With your legs still in
    that position, roll down onto your back,
    straighten the bottom leg, and extend it up
    to the ceiling for . . .

14. Supine Thread-the-Needle Pose
    And now, as though a stiff wind has just
    come along, topple over so that your top leg
    moves toward the opposite side for . . .

15. Supine Thread-the-Needle Twist
    Unwind and come back to where you were.
    Bring your knees into your chest and then
    rock up to . . .

16. Paripurna Navasana (Boat Pose)
    Cross your ankles and snap your fingers to
    make yourself smile and be a little playful.
    Rock over your feet into . . .

17. Phalakasana (Plank Pose)
    . . . and lower all the way down to the floor
    through . . .

18. Knees-Chest-Chin Pose
    . . . pushing up into . . .

19. Bhujangasana (Cobra Pose)
    Release the pose and push back into . . .

20. Adho Mukha Svanasana
    (Downward-Facing Dog)
    Bend your knees, look forward, and come to
    the top of your mat. Rise up into . . .

21. Urdhva Hastasana (Upward Salute)

Start all over again on the other side.

FINISHING POSE: Finish your practice with a
long, sweet Savasana (Corpse Pose).

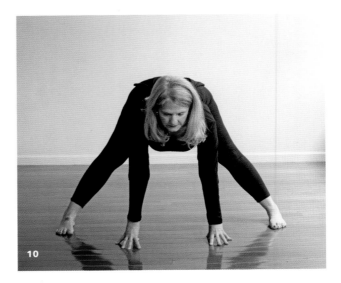

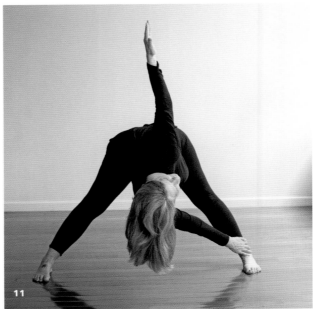

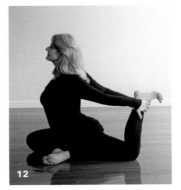

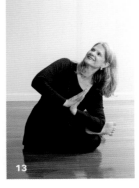

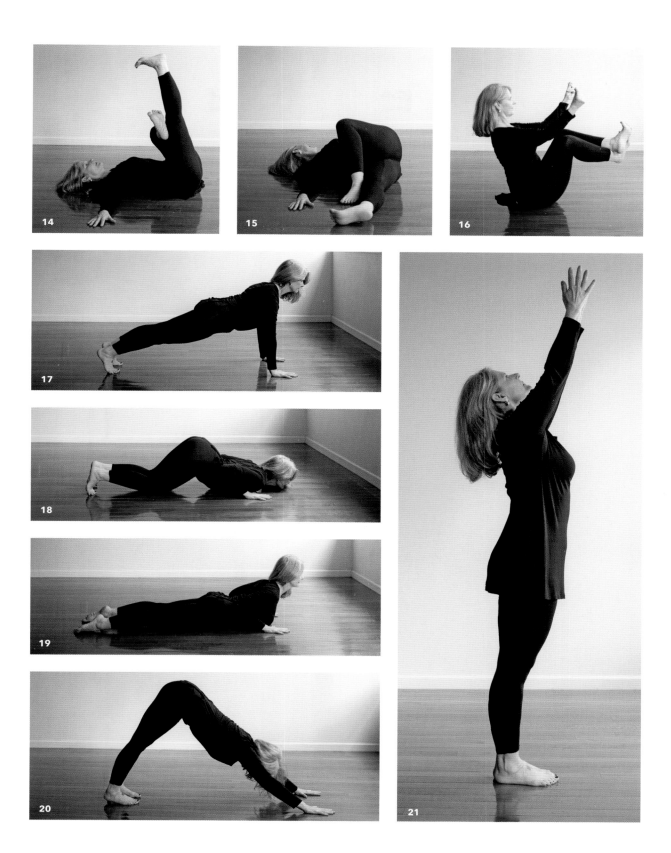

An Insight Yoga Practice

![lotus] SARAH POWERS

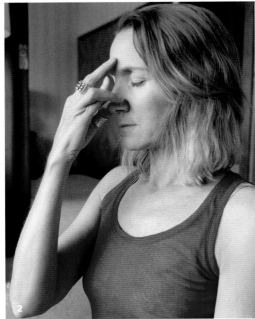

Wall need a place where we can sit down and listen, where we can bring the deeper teachings into our own bodies, at our own pace. We also need a place where we can move, strengthen, and enjoy our physicality. This Insight Yoga practice gives us both. If you have time, increase the 12 minutes of meditation to 24 minutes, the amount of time necessary to align the body and reset the nervous system.

BEGINNING: Sit in a comfortable position, with your eyes closed, for 3 to 5 minutes and ask yourself, "How am I feeling right now?" Vow to practice today with conscious intention by silently saying the following:

I vow now to develop mindful attention of this body, heart, and mind for my own and others' benefit. I appreciate its immeasurable value in how I live my life. I feel it is possible for me, as I learn to include all circumstances, feelings, and conditions.

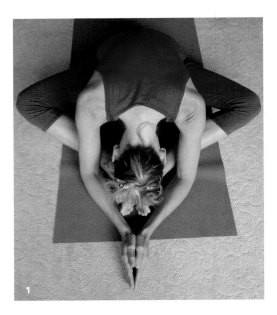

1. Butterfly Pose for 5 minutes
2. Nadi Shodhana Pranayama (Alternate Nostril Breathing variation) for 7 minutes
   - Inhale and exhale from the left nostril 3 full rounds
   - Inhale and exhale from the right nostril 3 full rounds
   - Inhale and exhale from both nostrils at once for 3 full rounds
   Focus: Breathe *in* vitality, breathe *out* and release mindlessness
3. Seated Meditation for 12 minutes (not pictured)
   - Breath concentration in the belly for 6 minutes
   - Mindfulness of the present moment for 6 minutes
4. Pelvic Circles
   - On the exhale 3 times in one direction, 3 times in the other direction, and then spend a few breaths quietly feeling the internal moves of the body

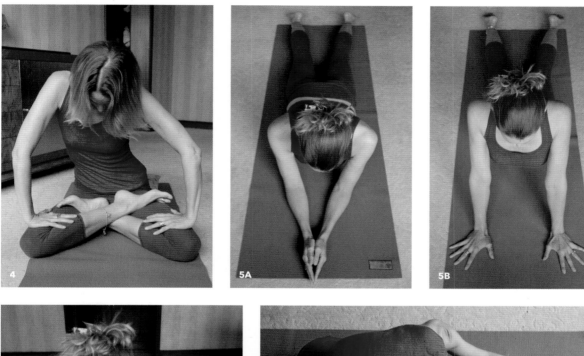

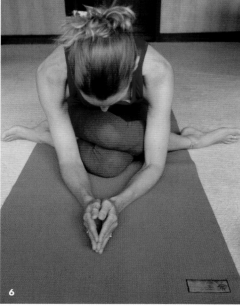

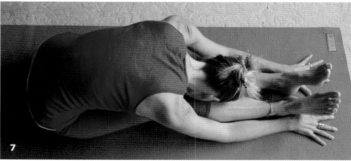

MIDDLE: Practice the next three yin poses, holding each one for 3 to 5 minutes.

5. Sphinx (A) or Seal (B) Pose
6. Shoelace Pose
7. Forward Bend

Move into the yang practice on the following spread, keeping the same *drishti* (focus) that you bring to your yin poses.

ROUND ONE: Stay in each pose for
5 full breaths.

1. Tadasana (Mountain Pose)
2. Urdhva Hastasana (Upward Salute)
3. Uttanasana (Standing Forward Bend)
4. Ardha Uttanasana
   (Standing Half Forward Bend)
5. High Lunge with right foot back
6. Chaturanga Dandasana
   (Four-Limbed Staff Pose)
7. Salabhasana (Locust Pose)
8. Bhujangasana (Cobra Pose)
9. Adho Mukha Svanasana
   (Downward-Facing Dog)
10. High Lunge with right foot forward
11. Anjaneyasana (Low Lunge)
    with arms up
12. Uttanasana (Standing Forward Bend)
13. Urdhva Hastasana (Upward Salute)
14. Tadasana (Mountain Pose)

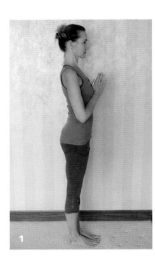

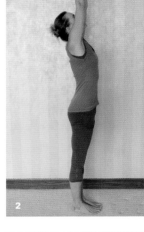

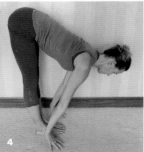

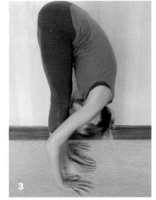

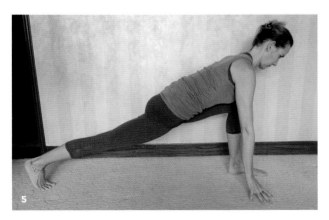

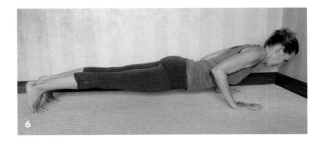

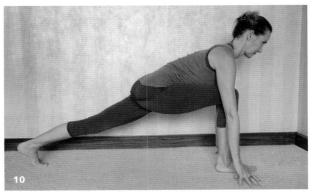

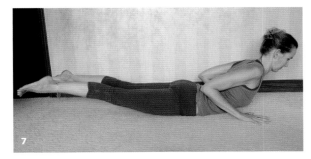

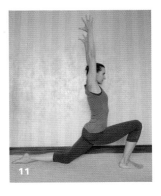

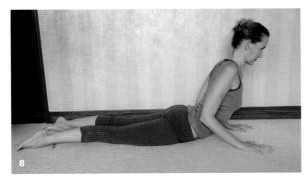

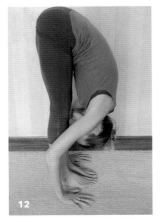

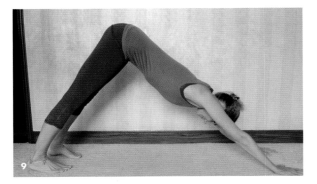

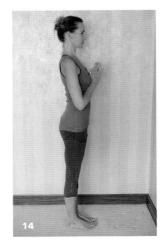

ROUND TWO: Stay in each pose for 5 full breaths.

1. Tadasana (Mountain Pose)
2. Urdhva Hastasana (Upward Salute)
3. Uttanasana (Standing Forward Bend)
4. Ardha Uttanasana (Standing Half Forward Bend)
5. High Lunge with hands on back
6. Anjaneyasana (Low Lunge) with backbend
7. Chaturanga Dandasana (Four-Limbed Staff Pose)
8. Salabhasana (Locust Pose)
9. Bhujangasana (Cobra Pose)
10. Adho Mukha Svanasana (Downward-Facing Dog)
11. Repeat pose 5 with right foot forward (not pictured)
12. Repeat pose 6 with right foot forward (not pictured)
13. Uttanasana (Standing Forward Bend)
14. Urdhva Hastasana (Upward Salute)
15. Tadasana (Mountain Pose)

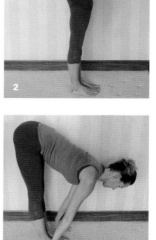
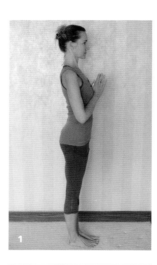
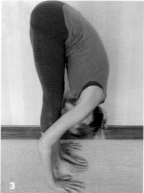
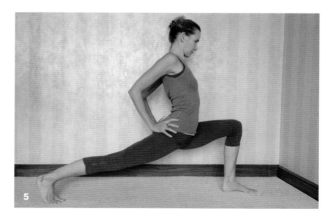

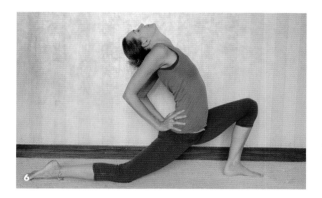

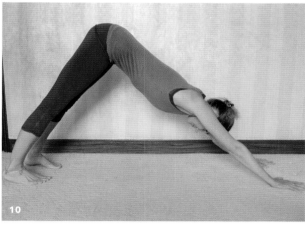

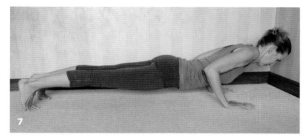

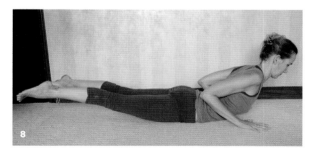

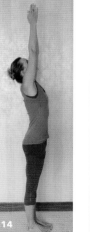

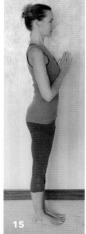

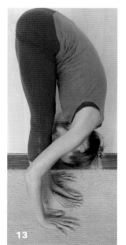

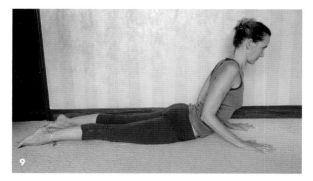

ROUND THREE: Stay in each pose for 5 full breaths.

1. Tadasana (Mountain Pose)
2. Urdhva Hastasana (Upward Salute)
3. Uttanasana (Standing Forward Bend)
4. Ardha Uttanasana
   (Standing Half Forward Bend)
5. High Lunge with twist
6. Anjaneyasana (Low Lunge) with twist
7. Chaturanga Dandasana
   (Four-Limbed Staff Pose)
8. Salabhasana (Locust Pose)
9. Bhujangasana (Cobra Pose)
10. Adho Mukha Svanasana
    (Downward-Facing Dog)
11. Repeat pose 5 with right foot forward
    (not pictured)
12. Repeat pose 6 with right foot forward
    (not pictured)
13. Uttanasana (Standing Forward Bend)
14. Urdhva Hastasana (Upward Salute)
15. Tadasana (Mountain Pose)

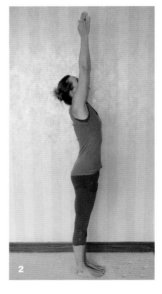
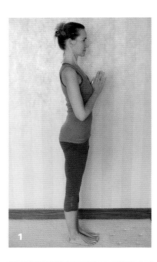
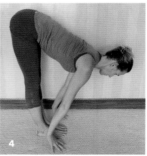
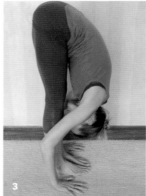
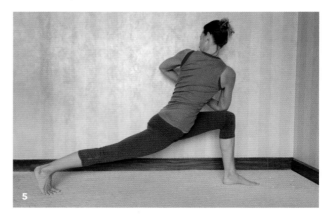

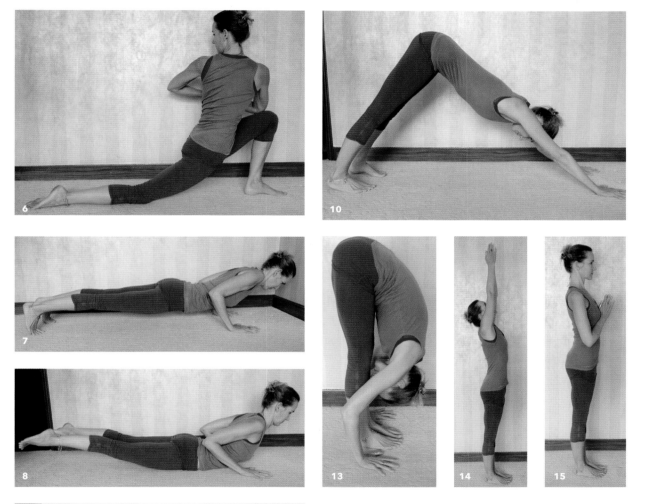

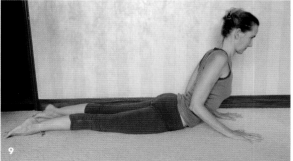

OPTIONAL STANDING SEQUENCE: Stay in each pose for 3 to 5 breaths.

1. Virabhadrasana I (Warrior I)
2. Virabhadrasana II (Warrior II)
3. Viparita Virabhadrasana (Reverse Warrior)
4. Utthita Parsvakonasana (Extended Side Angle)
5. Utthita Baddha Parsvakonasana (Bound Side Angle)
6. High Lunge
7. Adho Mukha Svanasana (Downward-Facing Dog)

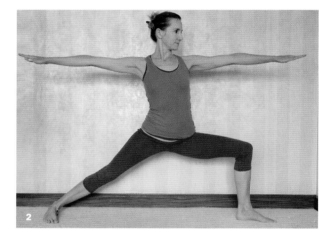

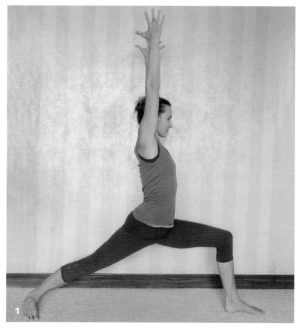

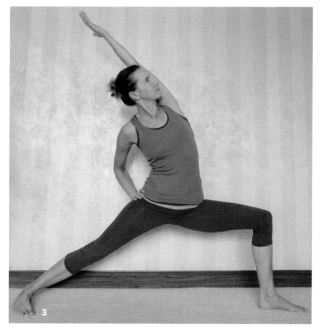

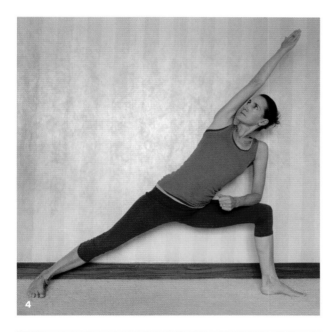

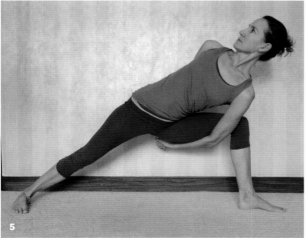

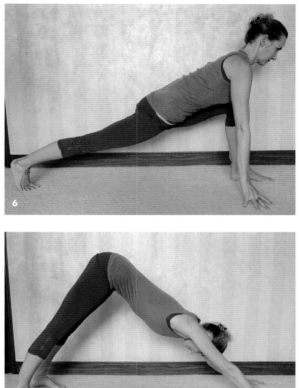

END: Rest in Savasana (Corpse Pose) and spend a few moments in Sukhasana (Easy Seated Pose) so you can end your practice with the intention to move into your day with gratitude and joy.

ADDITIONAL CONTRIBUTORS

In addition to the fifty-five wonderful practitioners profiled in the home stories section of this book, the following people also contributed their advice and expertise throughout other sections of *Yoga at Home*:

MAGDALINE ADHIAMBO found her heart's path through her work with students with special needs. As a yoga teacher with the Africa Yoga Project in Nairobi, Magdaline continues to study with Paige Elenson and Baron Baptiste.

ALICIA BARRY, a yoga teacher in Rhode Island, weaves mindfulness and yoga together into a profound healing modality for the body, mind, and spirit. She is known for her deeply transformative yin yoga classes.

BRENDA FEUERSTEIN is the director of Traditional Yoga Studies (TraditionalYogaStudies.com) and the author and coauthor of several books, including *The Yoga-Sutra from a Woman's Perspective*. She is the spiritual partner and wife of the late Georg Feuerstein, PhD (1947–2012).

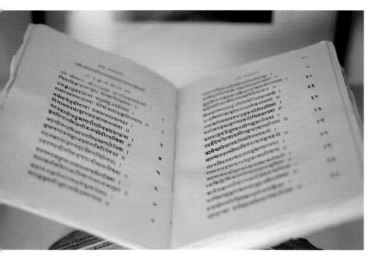

SUSAN KRAFT, a former dancer, approaches yoga as a tool, not only for physical health but also to enhance awareness and attention, and to steady the mind within the present moment. She teaches OM yoga in New York, New York.

DIANA KREBS needs daily yoga to stay on top of her job in Basel, Switzerland, where she's involved in geeky stuff like working on eGovernment strategies. Her seven-year-old son isn't interested in yoga, but he's her number one guru.

CYNDI LEE is the founder of OM yoga and an influential American yoga teacher. She is known for her dynamic and contemplative classes, creative sequencing, and smart and soulful teachings—all offered in a noncompetitive environment of goodness.

INSIYA RASIWALA-FINN, when not traveling around the world teaching workshops or leading Yoga, Ecology, and Surf Retreats, is at home in Vancouver, Canada, where she teaches challenging yet playful vinyasa classes. She can also be found on GaiamTV.com.

ROLF SOVIK is president and spiritual director of the Himalayan Institute, as well as the author of *Moving Inward: The Journey to Meditation* and coauthor of the award-winning *Yoga: Mastering the Basics*. You can find his writing and videos at YogaInternational.com.

FELICIA TOMASKO is a yoga teacher, ayurvedic practitioner, and the editor of *LA Yoga* magazine. She explores sacred energy through asana, pranayama, concentration, and relaxation. Her yin and vinyasa yoga classes can be found on YogaGlo.com.

BAS VAN KOLL is an award-winning creative director and strategic consultant who manages to find a bit of mental peace with his daily practice of vinyasa yoga and meditation amid the chaos of work, travel, and family activities.

RESOURCES

TOOLS

ONE-STOP SHOPPING

The following companies offer everything from eco-friendly mats, blocks, straps, and bolsters to eye bags, mat washes, and clothing:

Gaiam.com
HuggerMugger.com
Manduka.com
YogaProps.net
BarefootYoga.com

MATS AND ACCESSORIES

JadeYoga.com
Lululemon.com
ThreeMinuteEgg.com

SPECIALTY PROPS

Bhoga.com
Benches, wall units, chairs, and ergonomically designed "infinity blocks"

MightyBodyBand.com
Anti-gravity cross-training exercise device that includes swing, arm handles, and leg straps

YogaSwings.com
Omni swing with padded seat and foot stirrups

HarconYoga.com and **PinetreeYoga.com**
A full array of Iyengar wooden benches, backbenders, and trestlers

PRACTICE

This list of sources for information and online classes will help you focus your practice:

Yoga Journal (YogaJournal.com)
A great resource for advice, instructional pose videos, product recommendations, and so much more.

AimHealthyU.com
A health-focused website that includes *Yoga Journal*'s coursework around the business of yoga, a 10-hour yoga certification with Eddie Modestini, meditation, and more.

Other Online Asana Classes

YogaVibes.com
YogaAnytime.com
GaiamYogaStudio.com
GaiamTV.com/my-yoga

YogaGlo.com
YogaInternational.com
Pranamaya.com
JivamuktiYoga.com

CREDITS

PHOTOS

All photographs © Sarah Keough, except for the following:

© Rick Bern: pp. 162–165.
© Michael Chichi: pp. 94–97.
© Barb Colombo: pp. 24, 194–199, and 238.
© Fatih Demir: pp. 40–41 and 70–73.
© Audrey Derell: pp. 202–205.
© Geoffrey Ellis: pp. 60–63, 180–183, and 190–193.
© Daisy Erickson: pp. 208–209.
© John Bennett Fitts: pp. 1, 18, 106–109, and 144–147.
© Emily Gnetz: pp. 22 and 206–207.
© Stephen Langton Goulet: p. 17.
© Avsar Gulener: pp. 5 and 124–127.
© Kyrie Maezumi: p. 140.
© Yuri Manabe: pp. 14 (bottom left), 74–77, 86–87, and 176–179.
© Miko Matsumura: pp. 150–151.
© Tom McElroy: p. 141.
© Megan McIsaac: pp. 20–21, 37, 42–47, 82–85, and 98–101.
© James Mweu: pp. 128–129, 166–167, and 214–215.
© DJ Pierce: pp. 120–123.
© Dominique Pandolfi: pp. 56–59.
© Ty Powers: pp. 228–237.
© Angelique Sideris: p. 211.
© Mallika Singh: pp. 138–139.
© Bas Van Koll: pp. 10–11.

TEXT

Rolf Sovik's "Five Ways to Recharge Your Asana Practice" on page 39 originally appeared in the June/July 2004 issue of *Yoga International*. © 2004 Rolf Sovik. Adapted here with permission. Original can be found in its entirety at YogaInternational.com.

Shiva Rea's "Create Your Own Altar" on page 21 was adapted from her book *Tending the Heart Fire: Living in Rhythm with the Pulse of Life* (Sounds True, 2014). Adapted here with permission.

Patricia Walden's sample practice on page 156 originally appeared in the Summer 2013 issue of *Yoga International*. © 2013 Patricia Walden. Adapted here with permission. Original can be found as part of "Yoga for Cultivating Willpower" by Angela Wilson at YogaInternational.com.

ACKNOWLEDGMENTS

So many people came together to make *Yoga at Home* a reality. It would never have seen the light of day without the urging of Jim Muschett at Rizzoli International Publications and the support of Carin Gorrell, the editor in chief of *Yoga Journal*, who made our partnership especially sweet. Thank you both for your encouragement and your advice.

I'm beyond grateful to my collaborator, Sarah Keough, whose photos demonstrate her ability to dive deep into her subject matter. She captured the texture, quality, and quirky details of people's private lives with such care and affection that they gladly opened up their homes and hearts to us time and again.

Special thanks to Susi Oberhelman for creating a beautiful design, and to Candice Fehrman, my fabulous editor. Because of Candice's fierce attention to detail and her kind and generous attitude, I didn't even mind making those last inevitable changes.

Obviously this book would not have happened if it weren't for our incredible participants—dozens of yogis, artists, musicians, dancers, and business folks from all over the world—who shared their love of yoga, their homes, and their advice so freely. I bow to their generosity and wisdom.

Many thanks to Paige Elenson of the Africa Yoga Project; Terri Hinte, jazz publicist extraordinaire; Rolf Sovik of the Himalayan Institute; and all the contributing photographers who gracefully accepted our often impossible deadlines and delivered even beyond our expectations.

Sarah and I are indebted to and grateful for the loving attention and support of our families and friends: Ralph McGinnis, Jenifer Wanous, Jim Keough, Todd Holcomb, and Keith Yamashita.

And finally, I could never have written this book without the benefit of my practice, the wisdom of the ancient seers, and the generosity of my own teachers.

Published by Universe Publishing
A Division of Rizzoli International Publications, Inc.
300 Park Avenue South | New York, NY 10010 | www.rizzoliusa.com

© 2015 Universe Publishing | Text © 2015 Linda Sparrowe

Project Editor: Candice Fehrman | Book Design: Susi Oberhelman | Photo Editor: Sarah Keough

2015 2016 2017 2018 / 10 9 8 7 6 5 4 3 2 1

Printed in China | ISBN-13: 978-0-7893-2943-1 | Library of Congress Catalog Control Number: 2015933603